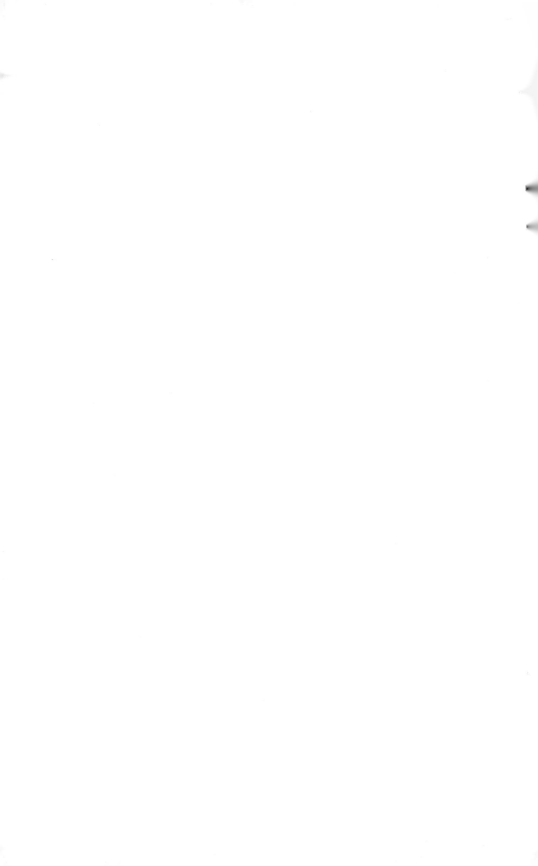

Health, Prevention and Economics

Health, Prevention and Economics

DAVID R. COHEN

*Reader,
Department of Management Studies,
Polytechnic of Wales*

and

JOHN B. HENDERSON

*Associate Research Fellow,
Health Economics Research Unit,
University of Aberdeen*

OXFORD   NEW YORK   TOKYO
OXFORD UNIVERSITY PRESS

Oxford University Press, Walton Street, Oxford OX2 6DP
Oxford New York Toronto
Delhi Bombay Calcutta Madras Karachi
Petaling Jaya Singapore Hong Kong Tokyo
Nairobi Dar es Salaam Cape Town
Melbourne Auckland
and associated companies in
Berlin Ibadan

Oxford is a trade mark of Oxford University Press

Published in the United States
by Oxford University Press, New York

© *D. R. Cohen and J. B. Henderson, 1988*

First published 1988
First published in paperback (with corrections) 1991

British Library Cataloguing in Publication Data
Cohen, David R.
Health, prevention and economics.
1. Health services. Economic aspects
I. Title   II. Henderson, John
338.4'73621
ISBN 0-19-261778-8
ISBN 0-19-262166-1 (Pbk)

Library of Congress Cataloging in Publication Data
Cohen, David R.
Health, prevention, and economics.
Includes index.
1. Medicine, Preventive—Economic aspects.
2. Medical economics.   I. Henderson, John B.   II. Title.
RA410.5.C63   1988   338.4'33621   88-17949
ISBN 0-19-261778-8
ISBN 0-19-262166-1 (Pbk)

Printed in Great Britain by
Dotesios Ltd., Trowbridge, Wiltshire

Preface

In most industrialized countries, expenditure on health care is rising at a much faster pace than increases in life expectancy and other indicators of health. Prevention is now commonly believed to be capable not only of producing greater increases in health than cure, but also of reducing the growth of health care expenditure. Many studies have therefore tried to show that prevention is cheaper than cure. It is easy to assume that this is all that economics has to offer, and there have been too few attempts to provide an overview to show, more generally, what economics can contribute to prevention.

We have tried to produce a text that is not overly specialized and that will appeal to the growing number of people with a professional interest in prevention and health. We believe that its arguments will be readily understood—even if not always completely agreed with—by a broad readership. We hope that it will be of particular interest and use to clinicians and other health care professionals, health policy makers, planners and managers, social scientists of many disciplines (including economics, of course), and to students of all these subjects.

Our experience of teaching on a wide variety of courses has guided our presentation of concepts and selection of examples, as well as reminding us of the need to minimize economists' jargon. In essence, we have tried to answer the twin questions:

1. How can economics and economists help in deciding upon priorities in the pursuit of health and the delivery of health-related activities?
2. What is the current state-of-the-art in economic approaches to prevention, that could inform the policy debate?

This book was conceived, planned, and partly written while we were research fellows at the Health Economics Research Unit (HERU) of the Department of Community Medicine, University of Aberdeen. We owe a great debt to many people there, but would like especially to mention two individuals. Professor Roy Weir, as head of the Department, *inter alia*, provided essential support for our activities there. Professor Gavin Mooney, former director of the HERU, acted above and beyond the call of duty, and even of friendship, in providing a sounding board for many of our ideas, and in reading and commenting on drafts of the text. We are pleased to acknowledge their help and to record our grateful thanks. We would also like to thank Margot, Annabel, and Sam for their forbearance during the writing process.

Naturally no one but ourselves bears any responsibility for any deficiencies or errors in the final text. It should be noted that although one of us (JBH) has since become an Economic Adviser to the Department of Health in London, this text does not necessarily represent their views.

Pontypridd   D.R.C.
March 1988   J.B.H.

Contents

1 Health, prevention and economics

1.1. Introduction

Prevention is currently fashionable, and in some ways this is unfortunate. Being fashionable is not conducive to rational debate: it disposes people to take up extreme positions. Some argue that prevention is always better than cure, that it alone in the realm of health care is deserving of greater priority, or even that curative care could be dispensed with if only greater efforts were devoted to prevention. Others argue that prevention is ineffective, that trying to change behaviour is futile and elitist, or that the sacrifices involved are too great. This book tries to stand back from heated arguments and unreasoned positions. Its aim is to help to inform the more tempered and rational debate that is replacing them.

A belief that prevention is cheaper than cure has led many to see prevention as a way of saving money, and economics as the discipline to highlight where these savings can be made. This shows a lack of understanding of both the objectives of prevention and of the role that economics can play in the pursuit of those objectives.

Economics provides the framework for considering issues of efficiency, and prevention will be shown to be amenable to economic appraisal. Economics also provides an analysis of preventive behaviour, and of the incentives that exist to prevent ill-health or to engage in activities that damage health. Such appraisal and analysis can produce essential information for devising, planning, implementing, and evaluating preventive programmes. If this book can increase the perception that economics offers another perspective, and one that is useful, we will be pleased. In this opening chapter we begin by clarifying the subject matter that is to be addressed.

1.2. What is health?

Everyone has an idea of what the term 'health' means, yet no one disputes that it is a difficult concept to define. A major reason for this is that health means different things to different people. Blaxter and Patterson (1982) provide the following example:

1

After I was sterilized I had a lot of cystitis, and a backache because of the fibroids. Then when I had my hysterectomy I had bother with my waterworks because my bladder had a life of its own and I had to have a repair . . . Healthwise I would say I'm O.K. I did hurt my shoulder—I mean, that is nothing to do with health, but I actually now have a disability . . . I wear a collar and take Valium, just the headaches—but I'm not really off work a lot with it.

Is this woman O.K. healthwise? That, of course, depends on one's point of view. As Twaddle (1974) has pointed out '. . . there is a wide consensus among medical people that illness is any state that has been diagnosed as such by a competent professional . . . Alternatively, there is a view that whoever feels ill should be regarded as sick.'

Health is a subjective concept as is evident when trying to measure, or even simply rank, different health states. Moreover, health is not only value-laden; it is multidimensional. For example, two of the many dimensions of health are pain and immobility. Other things being equal, more pain represents a lower state of health than less pain; more immobility a lower state of health than less immobility. But if one state involves more pain with less immobility than another it becomes impossible to determine objectively which is the better. The preferred state will vary between individuals according to such things as tolerance of pain or the importance of mobility in their work and social activities.

The meaning and measurement of health are not easy issues to deal with, yet they cannot be avoided. The main aim of prevention is the production of health. Chapter 4 will show that since the production of health involves the use of scarce resources that could have been put to other uses, it is essential that some means of measuring and valuing health be derived if the issue of efficiency is to be addressed. For the moment we will not try to provide solutions, but simply highlight the difficulties that arise. Of particular relevance is the elusive concept of *perfect health* and its distinction from *optimum health.*

There are interesting parallels between health and temperature. Cold is defined as the absence of heat, just as health is defined as the absence of illness. *Perfect cold* only exists at absolute zero. *Perfect health* is equally rare. Perfect health can be defined from a biological point of view as 'a state in which every cell of the body is functioning at optimum capacity and in perfect harmony with each other cell' (Twaddle 1974) or from a broader perspective as 'a state of complete physical, mental, and social well-being' (World Health Organization 1958).

Arguably, *perfect health* does not exist. However, most people do not concern themselves with the question of whether or not their current health state is perfect. Most people would not even choose to try to achieve perfect health for the simple reason that improvements in health status are not costless. Failure to recognize this simple fact largely explains why economists have been so slow in turning their attention to the whole area of health and health care. Fuchs (1972) pointed out that health issues had been ignored by economists because economics is essentially concerned with trade-offs (see Section 1.4) and economists had believed health to be so important that no individual would be willing to trade-off health for anything else. Examples can easily be found to demonstrate the falsity of that belief. Some individuals suffering the mild discomfort of a wart on their finger may well be unwilling to bear the costs of having it removed, while others may happily do so. Trade-offs exist; they also differ.

When the dimensions of time and uncertainty are introduced the falsity of the claim is even more evident. Smokers who are aware of the health hazards of smoking are trading-off the risk of future illness or death against their present satisfaction and pleasure. The same is true of people who willingly accept the risk of injury or death by crossing the road at a busy intersection rather than take the extra minute to walk to the pedestrian underpass down the road. As Cullis and West (1979) point out, 'Few people, if any, seek to maximize their health and life expectancy *per se*. To do so involves sacrificing opportunities to eat, drink, play games, drive, etc. that at the margin may be a greater source of utility than an additional (expected) minute or hour of life.'

The *costs* entailed in producing improvements in health need not be monetary, although money may be involved. Taking a safe job instead of a hazardous one might mean accepting lower wages, while living in good housing in a clean environment might mean paying higher rent. Having one's wart removed may mean paying the doctor, or paying the baby sitter to mind the children while being treated. What is less obvious is that factors not involving money also have associated costs since they involve a sacrifice of one form or another. Reducing the consumption of hazardous goods, such as cigarettes and alcohol, and eating less sugar and butter can involve the sacrifice of *pleasure*. Careful driving can mean longer journeys. Time spent in attending a screening clinic has a cost in that the benefits of other uses of that time are forgone. Hence, even if the individual is aware that these factors contribute to good health, he or she may not choose to accept the sacrifice if it is not justified by the benefits that would be derived from the improvement in health.

Thus *perfect* health is most unlikely to be the most desired state. Rather, the *optimum* state is that where the cost of any further improvement outweighs the value attached to that improvement. For each individual this optimum depends on perceptions of both the desirability of being healthy and the sacrifices involved in improving health. For the remainder of the book this notion of optimal health will be used.

1.3. What is prevention?

While the development of accurate and acceptable measures of health status may still be years away (Culyer 1983, Williams 1987), it is nevertheless possible to use the concept of theoretically measurable health status, and, in particular, the notion of a lifetime profile of health status, to help in clarifying what is meant by the term *prevention*. In principle, every individual can be viewed as being on some current level of health. This level may rise and fall through time and will ultimately end in death. There are four types of intervention through which the time profile of health status can be altered:

1. *Primary prevention* involves measures taken to prevent the onset of illness and injury. Primary prevention covers efforts to reduce the probability, severity, and duration of future illness and injury.
2. *Secondary prevention* involves measures to detect pre-symptomatic disease where earlier detection will mean more effective treatment. *Earlier* implies a stage before the individual would normally seek treatment, and usually before they would even be aware of disease.
3. *Tertiary prevention* involves measures to reduce the disability from existing illness and prevent it getting worse.
4. *Treatment and cure* cover activities to raise current levels of health status, from states of illness and injury.

Some clinicians go so far as to claim that secondary prevention is a misnomer because it does not prevent the onset of disease. This probably reflects their biological bias. From the individual's perspective, secondary prevention prevents the manifestation of illness so that their health, as they perceive it, does not deteriorate. This book adopts the perspective of the patient not the pathologist. Thus, following the definitions of health by Twaddle (1974) and WHO (1958) given in Section 1.2. above, disease is defined as 'imperfect harmony between cells', while illness is 'a perceptible state of physical, mental, or social malfunctioning'.

Tertiary prevention seeks to prevent a further fall in the health status profile after an initial fall (or an initial low level owing to a condition present from birth). It can therefore be hard, in practice, to distinguish tertiary prevention from cure. The distinction between tertiary prevention and cure is also blurred by any ambiguity about what is meant by health and illness.

Another area that does not fit tidily into the above taxonomy is *health promotion* which, although largely concerned with raising current health status, also promotes the message that raising current health status can reduce the risk of future illness. Health promotion is thus intrinsically linked with prevention and, in this book, is treated as a special form of primary prevention.

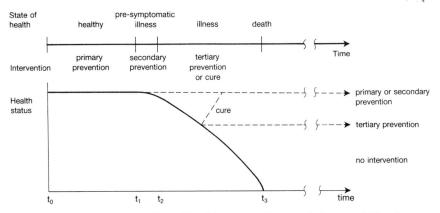

Fig. 1.1 Possible time paths of health status. *Source*: Cohen and Henderson 1983

Figure 1.1 shows one possible profile of health status over time and the alternatives associated with each of the four types of intervention. In the example, the individual is *healthy* between t_0 and t_1. The onset of pre-symptomatic illness arises at t_1, becomes symptomatic at t_2, and health status gradually declines until death occurs at t_3. In this illustration it is assumed that each type of intervention is 100 per cent effective and that the inevitable death occurs somewhere off the right side of the graph. Any of the interventions could be deemed *beneficial* if the area under the profile with the intervention is greater than the area under the profile without it. (Actually the benefit may also vary according to how soon it occurs, so a further refinement would be to consider the timing of rises and falls in health status. This is dealt with in Section 4.4.5.)

1.4. What is economics?

Efforts to raise the profiles of health status may involve a change in behaviour, greater use of health services, changing the environment, or some combination of these. Since they all have costs as well as benefits, preventing illness and improving health can be seen as a production process that has resource inputs and health outputs.

Paul Samuelson (1976) has defined economics as:

... the study of how men and society end up choosing, with or without the use of money, to employ scarce productive resources to produce various commodities over time and distribute them for consumption, now and in the future, among various groups and people in society. It analyses the costs and benefits of improving patterns of resource allocation.

Put more simply, economics is about the allocation of resources to production and the distribution of the output produced, bearing in mind that the ultimate end of economic activity is the consumption of output. Throughout this book economics is considered to be a *discipline*, by which we mean that the way of thinking is more important than particular techniques. The relevance of this discipline to prevention begins to become clearer when we look a little more closely at one of the key words in Samuelson's definition— *commodities*.

Commodities are the outputs resulting from productive processes. They may be goods or services, the only qualifications being that resources were used in their production and that they are of value. Health improvements can be viewed as commodities since they meet both of these conditions. Good health may be something with which most people are naturally endowed, but all efforts to improve this natural endowment, or to prevent it from falling, can be viewed as the production of the commodity health.

In the formal health care industry, health improvement is an output produced by combining various inputs, such as the time and skills of doctors and nurses, drugs, dressings, and operating theatres, with patients' own time. Chapter 9 shows how the commodity health can also be seen as something produced by individuals who combine various inputs such as healthy foods and exercise with their own time.

Viewed this way, health and prevention fit well into the framework of economics. The same way of thinking can be applied to this commodity as to the production and distribution of shoes or haircuts. Indeed it will be stressed that the production of health must compete for scarce resources with the production of other valued commodities.

Throughout this book, economic jargon is kept to a minimum, although some is useful. One piece of jargon that we make no attempt to avoid is *opportunity cost*. This concept is fundamental to answering the question, 'what is economics?'.

To most people the word *cost* suggests a sum of money. The cost of a television set is what you have to pay to acquire one. In economics, cost has a rather different meaning. Samuelson used the word *scarce* in his definition of economics to reflect the fact that resources are never sufficient to do everything that we would like to do. This does not imply that human beings are greedy, but states simply that there will never be enough resources to satisfy all human wants and desires. It also means that every time resources are committed to the production of one commodity, the opportunity to use those resources in the production of some other commodity is forgone. In other words a cost is incurred every time resources are used in one particular way; the cost being the value of the output that these resources could have produced had they been used in another way. Opportunity cost refers to the value of the sacrifice—the value of the benefit forgone.

Thus when an individual decides to be immunized against some disease, the *cost* is not only the price they may have to pay for the inoculation, but also such things as the value of their own time, since time spent travelling to and at the clinic means forgoing the benefits of using that same time for work or leisure.

There is one final word in Samuelson's definition that should be expanded upon before moving on. That word is *society*. Since economics is about making choices, it has to be asked who is to make these choices. In centrally planned economies, resource allocation decisions are made by committees who draw up 5- and 10-year plans. The values of committee members rule. In *perfect* free market economies, it is market forces alone that determine resource allocation. The values of individuals expressed through *consumer sovereignty* rule. In reality neither of these two extremes exists and a case for allocation by plan or by market can be made in particular circumstances under any type of political system. In any of these cases, though, some set of objectives must apply. Economics normally assumes that nobody's preferences are irrelevant, and that maximization of *social welfare* is the principal aim. This issue is discussed in more detail in Chapter 4.

1.5. A brief overview

Chapter 2 starts with a *macro* view, which examines the extent to which the health of nations determines the wealth of nations or *vice versa*. This is followed by seven chapters adopting a *micro* approach.

Chapter 3 explains the relevance of basic micro-economics to the study of prevention. Much of the simple theory of supply, demand, market failure, and the case for government intervention is equally applicable to some forms of prevention (for example, the supply of condoms or the demand for screening) as it is to other commodities. Consequently, while this book does not set out to be an economics textbook, it does contain some basic theory.

Chapter 4 explains the principles of economic appraisal. This provides the background to the case studies in primary and secondary prevention in Chapters 5 and 6. Chapter 7 considers the methodological issues and problems encountered in the empirical studies, explains how they were tackled, and describes good practice.

Because the focus of prevention is so often on the behaviour of individuals, Chapters 8 and 9 are both devoted to demand. The first of these presents empirical evidence of the effect of price, income, and other factors on the demand for prevention, while the second goes deeper into the theory behind preventive behaviour and presents an alternative to socio-psychological theories.

Chapter 10 returns to the broader view, with a discussion of the implications of earlier chapters for the construction of an overall prevention strategy. Expenditure on prevention in both the USA and the UK are identified and a *programme budget* for the UK is presented. The final chapter draws together the main conclusions, focusing on the notion of a coherent prevention policy.

2 Prevention and the economy

2.1. Introduction

Economic theory is conventionally divided into two parts; *macro-economics*, which is concerned with the economy as a whole, and *micro-economics*, which is concerned with specific decision-making units in the economy, such as the firm or the household. In the same way that macro-economics is about aggregates, the focus of *macro-prevention* is on reductions in morbidity and mortality generally, rather than on individual preventable outcomes or specific preventive measures. This chapter examines the relationship between macro-economics and macro-prevention.

On a global basis there is a clear relationship between the economies of nations and their levels of health. Grosse (1980) has estimated that as much as two-thirds of the variation in health status between nations may be explained by income differences. Of course, causality probably runs both ways: better health creates more wealth, and more wealth creates better health.

There are many reasons why increased income should lead to better health. With rising income comes better housing, a cleaner and safer environment, a more nutritious diet, and a host of other factors believed to improve health status. More income also means that there is more available for preventive services as well as other health and welfare programmes. However, more income can also mean an increase in the so-called *diseases of affluence* which are linked to a sedentary lifestyle and rich diet, motor vehicle accidents, and the consumption of alcohol and tobacco. Section 2.3 will look at the possible effects that changes in the economy as a whole have on health.

At the same time, it is argued that economic prosperity is itself largely determined by the health of the population. (Chapter 5 will show how increased productive output is a measurable benefit of health-creating programmes. Some of the theoretical models in Chapter 9 also link improved health with increased income.) It is hardly surprising, therefore, that developing nations are increasingly accepting the importance of investments in *human capital* as a means of bringing about economic development (Cumper 1983). In the US, Chang and Hsing (1980) have estimated that 8.3 per cent of US Gross National Product (GNP) is attributable to reductions in mortality rates since 1940. In the UK, one of the principal arguments in the debate which led to the setting up of a National Health Service (NHS) and the abolition of charges for health care, was that a healthier population would be more productive and would lead to greater economic prosperity. Section 2.4 will examine the effects of large-scale changes in health on the economy.

Establishing a relationship between national health and national wealth is one thing. Quantifying it and determining causality are quite another. While certain income-related variables such as housing and education may be known to be positively related to health status, the extent to which any changes in these variables create changes in health is unclear given the inevitable time lag between the initial and any resultant changes, and the many concurrent factors also affecting health. Equally, changes in health may precipitate changes in economic circumstances rather than *vice versa*. For example, the population of unemployed will be less healthy than the employed population since the former group will include those who are not working *because* of their poor health. Not surprisingly, the nature of the link between the state of the economy and the state of the nation's health is not well understood.

One area that appears to be producing some hard evidence of the link is the effect that unemployment has on health. Figure 2.1 shows the trends in mortality and unemployment rates for the UK over time. The only thing that can be said with certainty from this graph is that both rates fluctuate considerably over time. In order to answer the question, 'is there a connection?' a little background economic theory is required.

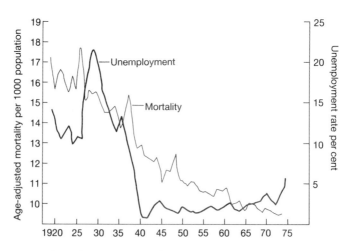

Fig. 2.1 Age-adjusted mortality and unemployment (UK 1922–1976). *Source*: Gravelle, Hutchinson, and Stern 1981.

2.2. The macro-economy and health

2.2.1. *Households, firms, and government*

This section simplifies macro-economic theory in order to make a few essential points. Economic theory is obviously more complex than is indicated here and interested readers will find a more detailed analysis in any elementary macro-economics textbook.

One measure of economic well being is *Gross Domestic Product* (GDP) which represents the value of all the (final) goods and services produced in an economy in one year. The long-term trend of GDP is normally upward, meaning that economic growth is a long-term feature of most economies. In the short term there are fluctuations around the trend.

Downward fluctuations mean that the economy is not producing all that it is capable of producing. These periods are associated with unemployment—i.e., labour that is available and willing to work but cannot find jobs. Why does this happen?

The economy can be described in simple terms as a *circular* system as shown in Figure 2.2.

The economy comprises two principal sectors; households and firms, with a third sector, government, playing the role of intermediary. Concentrating on the two principal sectors we see that firms, which may be privately or publicly owned, demand labour (as well as other productive services) from households,

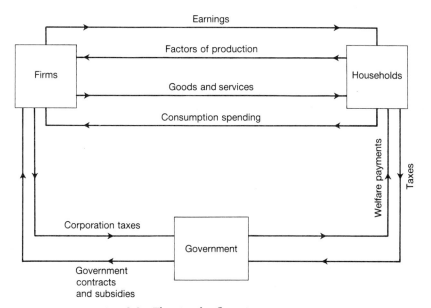

Fig. 2.2 The circular flows in an economy.

and that this labour is used to produce goods and services. In return, households demand goods and services from the firms for consumption. Together these represent the circular flow of physical resources.

At the same time there is a flow of money between these two sectors, with households paying firms for the goods and services they consume, and firms paying households wages (and other returns) for their labour (and other services). The government takes a share of the money flow in the form of taxes which can then be re-distributed as welfare benefits to households or as subsidies to firms.

In addition to its distributional role, government demands goods and services from firms; for example, by hiring construction firms to build roads. In this simple model the amount that firms produce depends upon the demands for goods and services from households, and the demands (on behalf of households) from government (i.e. public expenditure). In turn, the amount of labour that firms demand depends upon the amount of output they produce.

If the demand for goods and services falls, firms produce less. They then demand less labour which causes unemployment to rise. The government can increase demand by increasing public expenditure. It can demand roads, hospitals, sewerage systems, public housing, schools—which are built by firms using labour. It can also increase the demand for labour directly by instructing public corporations to employ more teachers, nurses, police officers, environmental health officers, etc. Thus government can reduce unemployment. When employment falls, however, tax revenue from earnings also falls. So where does the government get the money to pay for all this expansion in demand? Put simply, it can borrow it or it can print it.

Unfortunately, there are repercussions from either of the above. Government borrowing displaces some private investment out of the pool of savings and printing money is inflationary. If keeping inflation down and not crowding out private investment are also priorities, then the measures available to reduce unemployment will be limited.

The essential points from this simplified analysis are that:

1. Demands upon firms fluctuate and this is a major cause of fluctuating employment.
2. Governments try to varying degrees to smooth the fluctuations and prevent unemployment rising too much.
3. The extent to which they try to manage unemployment is determined by the importance of this objective *vis-à-vis* other government priorities, and the perceived extent of their capacity to succeed (matters of lively controversy between the Monetarist and the Keynesian schools).
4. No matter what their commitment to smoothing the fluctuations, governments never completely succeed because their information is never completely up-to-date. (Again, the Monetarists and Keynesians disagree on the importance of this factor.)

2.2.2. *Macro-economic cycles and health: the connections?*

2.2.2.1. The effect on health of government spending Many of the things that the government spends money on would be expected to affect health. Spending on roads and traffic police should reduce accidents; spending on sewerage, refuse collection, housing, and on reducing environmental pollution should reduce the spread of disease; spending on education should improve knowledge of how to be healthier; and, of course, spending on health services should improve health. If spending on these factors rises, then morbidity and mortality rates should fall. If the government spends more on these, in response to unemployment, then unemployment, morbidity, and mortality should fall together.

2.2.2.2. The effect on health of unemployment Unemployment means less wages. Decreased incomes mean that less will be spent on all goods, including hazardous goods such as alcohol and cigarettes, and decreased consumption of such hazardous goods will reduce morbidity and mortality. At the same time most goods which are considered to be health promoting are also 'normal' (as opposed to 'inferior') in the sense that a fall in income will cause a fall in demand. There are thus two counteracting effects of decreased income.

An alternative connection between unemployment and ill-health is more direct. This hypothesis is that trying to find a job and failing to do so is stressful. Stress may lead directly to mental ill-health or suicide, or, indirectly, to illnesses such as heart disease.

2.2.2.3. The effect on the economy of increased health One way of describing 'healthiness' is in terms of the number of healthy days available for work or leisure. Within this framework an increase in health means a greater supply of labour, and a greater supply of labour, without an increase in the demand for labour, means higher unemployment. Hence reductions in mortality may lead to absolute increases in unemployment, although reductions in morbidity may lead only to a switch from being 'off-sick' to being 'unemployed'. There are, therefore, many connections in theory, but are they important in practice? The next two sections address this question from two angles.

2.3. Could macro-economic management prevent ill-health?

The answer to this question depends on two issues:

1. Whether macro-economic variables such as income, government expenditure and unemployment can be *managed*—i.e. controlled by government.
2. Whether macro-economic variables such as income, government expendi-

ture, and unemployment reduce, increase, or have no net effect upon health.

The first issue is a question of both economics and politics. From the economic perspective, the extent to which such economic variables are controllable is a matter of controversy with economists of the 'new classical' school denying that they can be accurately managed and most others, especially the Keynesians, arguing that they can be. Whether or not there are more important competing priorities is a question of politics. The second issue—whether economic variables affect health—is of greater concern here.

2.3.1. The evidence 'for'

The issue of whether macro-economic variables affect health has been investigated by many, but most famously by Brenner (1967 and subsequent) who claims to have found a relationship between macro-economic variables, mortality, and morbidity. Brenner's studies suggest that increases in unemployment have increased mortality and morbidity, and that periods of rapid growth in incomes have had the same effect (Brenner 1967, 1973, 1977). In his studies of the US, Brenner claimed that a 1 per cent rise in unemployment would lead to 36 886 deaths in the following 6 years.

In his study of trends and fluctuations in GNP and mortality in England and Wales, Brenner (1979) claimed that:

(1) the GNP trend was up, the mortality trend down;
(2) unemployment was correlated with mortality—i.e. slowed down the trend;
(3) rapid rises in GNP (income per capita) were correlated (weakly) with mortality;
(4) government welfare expenditure as a proportion of all government expenditure was correlated with reduced infant and child mortality.

2.3.2. The evidence 'against'

Brenner's work has been subject to much criticism mainly on methodological grounds. Perhaps the most severe criticism came from Gravelle, Hutchinson, and Stern (1981) who identified four categories of flaw in Brenner's approach.

2.3.2.1. *The data*   Results are only as good as the data upon which they are based, and Brenner's data had several faults. For example, Brenner used disposable (after tax) income rather than GNP per capita as the income variable. Thus in Brenner's model, if government were to raise taxes to fund increased expenditure on health, the expected effect would be a *reduction* in health.

Another variable which came under criticism was 'government welfare expenditure as a percentage of total government expenditure'. Use of this variable implies that if government were to increase spending on road safety, the expected effect would be a reduction in health.

2.3.2.2. *Omissions* Brenner's model did not take into account many of the other important factors that contributed to changes in morbidity and mortality over the period in question. For example, no account was taken of the introduction of antibiotics, of better nutrition, or of the role of education.

2.3.2.3. *Mis-specified time lags* While estimating time lags between cause and effect is never an easy matter, Gravelle, Hutchinson, and Stern argued that Brenner got it backwards. Whereas Brenner assumed that the effect of higher unemployment on morbidity and mortality increased for a few years then declined, Gravelle, Hutchinson, and Stern re-estimated the model and found that the effect declined then increased.

2.3.2.4. *Robustness* The relationships which Brenner claimed to have found for the period 1936–1970 gave incorrect predictions for the period 1970–1978.

Another major problem concerned the inability to establish causation even if correlation could be demonstrated. For example, did unemployment cause disease, did disease cause unemployment, or both? Did unemployment cause stress which caused death or did stress lead to unemployment, which led to poverty, which caused death?

After replicating Brenner's model for England and Wales, Gravelle, Hutchinson, and Stern concluded:

Our results and criticisms, although casting considerable doubt on Brenner's results for Britain, do *not* mean that unemployment has no adverse health effects. Indeed it is plausible that such effects do exist—but there is as yet, no evidence which can be used to estimate their magnitude, timing, and form. (p. 678)

Attempts by other economists to replicate Brenner's model have also produced little support for his conclusions. McAvinchey (1982) used lagged unemployment and income as possible causal variables on mortality in Scotland between 1950 and 1978. Though establishing a weak link, especially for the over 35 age group, McAvinchey found the model and results were quite sensitive to the estimation method used.

Also looking at Scotland, Forbes and McGregor (1987) found little evidence to support the hypothesis that mortality was linked to unemployment, except in the case of mortality from lung cancer and ischaemic heart disease in older males. Even then the association only held in the short term.

In his review of the work in this area, Wagstaff (1985) concluded:

The time series methodology may yet yield convincing evidence at a macro-level that the social costs of unemployment and rapid growth include premature deaths. At the moment, however, there is no such convincing evidence. . . . In the meantime, it would be most unwise for policy makers to go on accepting Brenner's results as readily as has apparently been the case hitherto. (p. 995)

2.3.3. The debate continues; some more evidence 'for'

One problem with all the foregoing studies is that because the connections between unemployment and health are multiple and complex it is difficult to disentangle the various effects using data at the aggregate level. Controlled prospective studies of individuals would give much better evidence.

Such evidence has been provided by a few studies. Stafford, Jackson, and Banks (1980) measured the mental health of a group of children before and after leaving school. They found that those who found jobs after leaving school had better mental health than those who did not. Moreover, the mental health of the unemployed improved when they found jobs, while that of the employed worsened if they lost their jobs. Such findings add much weight to the evidence that unemployment causes mental ill-health and ultimately, in some cases, suicide.

Perhaps the best evidence comes from the study by Moser, Fox, and Jones (1984) which used the UK Census of Population as its data base. From a longitudinal study of 1 per cent of the total census population carried out by the Office of Population Census and Surveys (OPCS), the authors focused on those men aged 15–64 who were seeking work in the week preceding the 1971 census. Their main results can be summarized under four headings:

2.3.3.1. *Excess mortality*   The mortality of these men in the period 1971–1981 was higher than would be expected from the death rate for all men in the study, even after adjusting for socio-economic circumstances thus lending support to Brenner's conclusions.

2.3.3.2. *Stress leads to suicide*   Their results supported previous studies which had suggested that stress accompanying unemployment could be associated with increased suicide rates.

2.3.3.3. *Raised mortality is not due to illness causing unemployment*   The trend in overall mortality and the pattern by causes of death implied that it was unlikely that excess mortality was due to the men having become unemployed because of ill-health. In other words the raised mortality was not due to initial poor health in this group.

2.3.3.4. *Wives of unemployed men also had raised mortality*   The mortality rates of the wives of the unemployed men were raised even after adjusting for socio-economic circumstances.

The authors repeated their study for the period 1981–1983 using the OPCS 1 per cent longitudinal study of the 1981 census population, to see if the results would be similar during a period of much higher unemployment than was the case in the previous study (Moser, Goldblatt, Fox, and Jones 1987). All of the above four findings were repeated. There is thus strong evidence of an association between unemployment and ill-health, and the direction of causation does not appear to be from ill-health to unemployment.

The possibility that the real cause is something else, however, cannot be ruled out. It could, for example, be that the real cause is poverty. However, even if the real cause is poverty, the solution would be the same; to increase government spending to alleviate poverty and raise income. The conclusion would seem to be that macro-economic policy could be used to prevent premature mortality and ill-health.

2.4. Could more prevention harm the macro-economy?

Some of the most important causes of years of life lost are to a significant extent preventable (see Figs 10.1 and 10.2). If they were prevented there would be more people around living longer lives. What would the effect of this be? We begin by looking at the prospects for prevention.

2.4.1. *Macro-prevention*

McKeown (1979) has examined the reasons for the modern rise of population. He examined the causes of deaths over the last 300 years in England and Wales and found that the main reason for the decline in mortality rates, especially in the nineteenth century, was the reduction in communicable diseases. The main effect of this was to increase life expectancy for infants and children. Similar effects have been found for the US.

The current situation is considerably different. Apart from sudden infant death syndrome and congenital malformations, the main effects of reducing the preventable causes of years of life lost would be among adults. Moreover, apart from causes such as motor vehicle and other accidents, suicide, and homicide, a large part of the effect would be on adults aged over 60 years.

But what is the potential for macro-prevention? One way of assessing the feasibility of reducing preventable mortality is to review the prospects for prevention for each cause separately. This has been done in the UK by Doll (1983). For some causes the prospects are quite clear. For example,

The avoidance of smoking would alone reduce the mortality from all cancers by about a third (including avoidance of not only the large majority of cancers of the mouth, throat, and lung, but also a substantial proportion of the deaths attributed to cancers of the bladder, kidney, and pancreas). It would almost eliminate chronic obstructive lung disease and the complications of peripheral vascular disease, would reduce the age specific mortality from aortic aneurysm by at least three quarters and the mortality from myocardial infarction by about a quarter, and would probably lead to a small reduction in perinatal mortality in the poorer socioeconomic groups. (p. 448)

For other causes the prospects are far less clear.

Table 2.1 shows eight major causes of death in the US and the associated risk factors. In every case prevention can reduce the mortality rates, but the amount by which each can be reduced is difficult to specify. The recent reductions in coronary heart disease in the US, however, show that the scope for macro-prevention is large.

Another way of assessing the potential for macro-prevention is to compare disease-specific mortality rates across countries, although there might be good geographical or genetic reasons why it might be difficult to draw valid conclusions from this. For example Table 2.2 shows that the UK mortality rate for lung and throat cancer in males is 60 per cent higher than that in the US, and almost five times that for Portugal.

If it is accepted that macro-prevention is possible, what effect might it have on the national economy? To answer this question requires consideration of some more theory.

2.4.2. *Macro-economic modelling*

Macro-economic modelling seeks to predict the effects of changes in one part of the economy on the rest by modelling the relationships between the various

Table 2.1   Major causes of deaths in the United States, 1977

Cause	Major risk factors
Heart disease	Smoking, hypertension, elevated serum cholesterol
Malignant neoplasms	Smoking, worksite carcinogens
Stroke	Hypertension, smoking, elevated serum cholesterol
Accidents (other than motor vehicle)	Alcohol
Influenza and pneumonia	Vaccination status
Motor vehicle accidents	Alcohol, no seat belts, speed
Diabetes	Obesity
Cirrhosis of the liver	Alcohol abuse

Source: US Department of Health and Human Services 1980

Table 2.2 Malignant trachea-, bronchio-, and lung-neoplasm mortality rates in males, 1980 (selected countries)

Country	Rate per 100 000 population
Australia	55.3
Belgium	112.8
Canada	59.6
France	58.0
Japan	27.0
Portugal	23.1
United Kingdom	111.2
United States	68.4

Source: Organization for Economic Co-operation and Development 1985

components. For example, based on the relationships derived from the study of previous changes, a model could predict the effect of a reduction in the rate of income tax on labour supply, labour demand, employment, output, income, inflation, etc. The prediction would be based on the effect of the change as it worked its way around the system as shown in Fig. 2.2. Macro-economic models are used by governments to help them calculate the effects of economic policy changes, before they commit themselves to particular new policies.

The implications of the previous section are that the main effect of a macro-prevention effort would be an increase in the supply of labour, and also an increase in the number of people of post-retirement age. The effect of an increase in the aggregate supply of labour can be depicted as in Figure 2.3. (A fuller explanation of supply and demand curves is given in Chapter 3.)

This diagram shows an increase, i.e. an outward shift, in the labour supply schedule. The effect is seen to be an increase in hours worked, but also a fall in wage rates. In this diagram the demand for labour is assumed to be insufficiently responsive to changes in wage rates so that total wages paid decrease (from $W_1 \times H_1$—the area under the W_1 line—to $W_2 \times H_2$—the area under the W_2 line).

If the total amount of wages paid decreases, then government receipts of income taxes will also fall. If tax receipts fall then welfare benefits fall. If incomes fall then consumer demand falls. If consumer demand falls then output falls. If output falls the demand for labour falls, and so on.

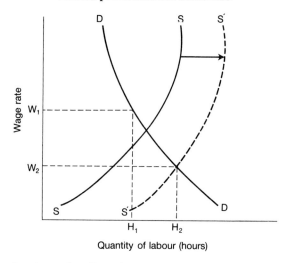

Fig. 2.3 The effect of a shift in the supply of labour.

This chapter now turns to what effects macro-prevention may have on the economies of the US and the UK.

2.4.3. *Macro-economics of prevention in the US*

In an ambitious study Gori and Richter (1978) have shown the effect that a macro-prevention effort could have on the US economy. If the US could achieve the mortality rates from preventable diseases of the countries with the second lowest rates in the industrialized world (on the grounds that the lowest might be an aberration) then the number of premature deaths avoided would be as in Table 2.3.

The authors then applied these prevention rates to the US population age- and sex-specifically, although it should be noted that their forecasts assume no other changes. As a result they were able to indicate, for example, that life expectancy at birth would increase by 5 years, at age 30 by 3 years, and at age 60 by 2 years. These age-specific increases were then put into the 'Wharton Econometric Forecasting Model'. The initial predictions were bleak, showing for example that GNP would fall by $106 billion (1972 prices) and unemployment would rise by 7 million within twenty years.

They tried an alternative set of population estimates, based on the assumption that rather than being achieved overnight, the increase in population would be phased over 25 years. The results were less depressing, showing, for example, that GNP would increase by $20 billion (1972 prices) and unemployment would rise by only 1 million within twenty years.

Table 2.3 Mortality from the five major causes (1973) and prevention potential calculated by comparing US mortality rates with next-to-the-lowest rates among industrialized countries

Causes	No. of deaths	Percentage of total mortality	Prevention potential (%)
Major cardio- vascular-renal diseases	1 012 341	51	39
Malignant neoplasms	351 055	18	25
Accidents, motor vehicle and other	115 821	6	38
Respiratory diseases	92 267	5	17
Diabetes mellitus	38 208	2	63
All other	363 311	18	—

Source: Gori and Richter 1978

As the US population would in any case grow during this time, the authors might have expressed their findings more appropriately in GNP per capita terms. Nevertheless, the conclusions to be drawn are that a sudden dramatic increase in labour supply would probably harm the US economy, but a gradual increase in population by increased preventive efforts would probably do little harm.

It must be remembered that such forecasts 20 years into the future (as it was then) are unreliable because they assume no other changes; an assumption that becomes increasingly unrealistic. Also GNP is only a measure of tangible and market-priced resource consequences. It does not include unpriced benefits such as increases in leisure time, nor intangible benefits such as less pain and suffering from illness. (Chapter 4 spells out the benefits of reduced morbidity and mortality more fully.) Hence the total benefits may be understated by the GNP measure.

On the other hand some preventive measures, such as reduced speed limits (see Section 5.2.8) would decrease available leisure rather than increase it. Others, such as reducing smoking, may reduce satisfaction (utility). Yet others, such as reducing stress, may increase the satisfaction from all consumption.

Other caveats include the fact that it is not known how policy makers would react. The model assumes that taxes would be increased to redistribute to those in the post-retirement age bracket. But would policy makers necessarily want to do this? Gori and Richter's results must therefore be seen as speculative, but the observation that too sudden an increase in macro-prevention may be harmful to the economy should not be overlooked.

2.4.4. *Macro-economics of prevention in the UK*

There is no equivalent of the Gori and Richter study for the UK. Nevertheless, it is possible to infer effects for potential years of working life lost and the effects of a larger labour force on the UK economy.

Table 2.4 shows that a reduction in mortality rates for ischaemic heart disease by 20 per cent in England and Wales would increase years of potential working life by about 48 000 person years (39 000 for men and 8500 for women). If motor vehicle traffic accident mortality rates were reduced by 20 per cent, the increase would be approximately 20 000 years for men and over 5600 for women.

Ermisch (1983) has estimated the effects of different population growth rates on forecasts of employment and unemployment up to the year 2001. He used a pessimistic assumption of growth rates in employment of -0.04 per cent per annum, based on UK experience in the period 1965–1979 and an optimistic assumption of 0·4 per cent per annum, based on the UK experience in the period 1956–1960. Results are shown in Table 2.5.

It can be seen that higher fertility rates have the effect of producing higher unemployment levels. Ermisch concludes that:

The size of the increase in Britain's potential labour supply poses an unemployment problem of huge dimensions under most feasible macro-economic policies. (p. 169)

Table 2.4   Years of working life lost due to mortality from certain causes, England and Wales 1985

Cause of death	Years of working life lost* (thousands)
Cancer of trachea, bronchus, and lung	69.8
Cancer of female breast	60.3
Ischemic heart disease	238.0
Other heart disease and hypertension	43.1
Cerebrovascular disease	62.3
Bronchitis, emphysema, and asthma	27.5
Other diseases of the respiratory system	25.8
Motor vehicle traffic accidents	122.5

* = Males and females aged 15–64
Source: Office of Population Censuses and Surveys 1987

Table 2.5 Changes in unemployment GB

	1991–96 Fertility		1996–2001 Fertility	
	Low	High	Low	High
Unemployment level increase, thousands				
optimistic	− 340	− 280	− 330	+ 70
pessimistic	+ 230	+ 290	+ 245	+ 645

Note: Optimistic = growth in employment of 0.4 per cent p.a. Pessimistic = growth in employment of − 0.04 per cent p.a.
Source: Ermisch 1983

The same conclusion would apply to increases in labour supply achieved by macro-prevention. A possible consequence could be higher unemployment and lower average incomes.

2.5. Conclusions

This chapter has shown that, although there is evidence that the national economy and national health are related, it is by no means easy to identify the direction of cause and effect. Governments can control the economy to some extent, but will government control of the economy be preventive? On the one hand it can be, since much government spending will be on goods and services that will directly increase health. On the other hand any reductions in unemployment that government economic policy brings about will only be preventive if unemployment is a cause of morbidity and mortality. On present evidence it is not possible to say whether or not it is. The *tentative* conclusion would be that unemployment does in fact cause increased morbidity and mortality. Macro-economic policies which reduce unemployment are, there-fore, probably preventive.

But what effect will macro-prevention have on the macro-economy? Again it is hard to answer this question. It must be emphasized though, that prevention in the past largely meant reducing infant and childhood mortality. While there is still much scope for prevention today, current preventive measures largely mean either extending the lives of retired people or increasing the labour supply for which there may be no work. It would seem that a highly successful prevention policy which produced immediate and dramatic results could adversely affect the economy.

This does not mean that an ambitious prevention policy is necessarily a bad thing. It would be dangerous to draw such general conclusions from an analysis which looks only at the tangible, market-priced, resource consequences of prevention and ignores all of the intangible benefits such as less pain, grief, and suffering. Such a conclusion would be analogous to a cost–benefit analysis which concluded on a similar basis that all programmes of care for the elderly or the mentally handicapped should not be pursued. The fact that societies do care for these client groups shows that the implied value of their lives is clearly positive.

It is important that more evidence be provided to show how macro-prevention affects the macro-economy, but the ultimate desirability of macro-prevention will not be decided by this evidence alone.

3 Consumers, producers, and government

3.1. Introduction

Among other things, micro-economic theory attempts to explain consumers' demand, producers' supply, and whether or not there is any justification for the government intervening in the freely made choices of consumers or suppliers. This chapter concentrates on the last of these issues.

Consider the following example: Joe Brown has just bought a new motorcycle and is now considering the pros and cons of buying (and wearing) a crash helmet. Wanting to be a rational informed consumer, he gathers all the evidence on motorcycle safety, determines the statistical risk of injury or death with and without a helmet, and, after also determining the types of injuries possible and their consequences, decides not to wear a helmet. In many countries such a decision is considered unacceptable. If an individual will not voluntarily demand a helmet, the law can, and in most places does, compel him or her to wear one. But why?

This chapter considers the pros and cons of interfering with the freely made choices of consumers and producers. Since analysis of the role of the state requires some knowledge of how the system operates in the absence of any form of government intervention, this chapter begins with an explanation of how unregulated markets can, in theory, solve the two main problems in economics—how to allocate resources to the production of a range of commodities and how to distribute those commodities for consumption. The next section picks apart those assumptions necessary for the market model to work in the way described and explains how government intervention can be justified when such market imperfections exist.

Since the market for cigarettes contains many of the attributes which can lead to market failure, it will be used as an illustration to highlight the role for market intervention. The reader should be able to apply the principles from this example to other situations.

3.2. The free-market solution to allocation and distribution

Economic theory can demonstrate that, given certain conditions, unregulated markets will solve the twin economic problems of allocation of resources and distribution of output. Economists of all political colours agree with this. The controversy arises in analysing these 'certain conditions'.

3.2.1. *Supply, demand, and market equilibrium*

The DD curve in Figure 3.1 is a 'demand curve' and reflects the fact that at lower prices a greater quantity is demanded by consumers than at higher prices. The principle behind this is that consumers derive satisfaction or utility from consumption, and that beyond some point the extra utility yielded by any additional unit of the good declines. Because utility determines willingness to pay, a consumer will be willing to pay more for the earlier units than the later units. There is, however, a common price for all units so the consumer will demand only the earlier units when price is high, but will demand a greater amount when the price is lower.

The SS curve is a 'supply curve'. It shows that at higher prices producers have an incentive to produce larger quantities of the good than at lower prices.

Both curves are drawn up for a 'given state of the world'. They show how the quantities demanded and supplied vary over different prices with all other things constant. If any of these other things, such as tastes and preferences, prices of other goods, or costs of production change, then these curves may have to be redrawn.

The DD and SS curves show the quantities which consumers will demand and producers will supply for all possible prices. Figure 3.1 also shows what the actual price and quantities supplied and demanded will be. If price is above P(e), say at P(1), then the amount which producers supply Q(1) is greater than the amount which consumers demand Q(2). With more of the good on the

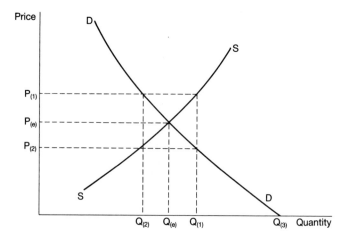

Fig. 3.1   Supply and demand curves.

market than can be sold there will be pressure on price to fall. If price is below P(e), say at P(2), then the amount which producers wish to supply Q(2) is less than the amount which consumers wish to buy Q(1). Consumers will be chasing an insufficient quantity of goods to satisfy them all, so there will be pressure on price to rise.

The only price and quantity that can be sustained without any pressure for change, are P(e) and Q(e). These are the *equilibrium* price and quantity, and the market is in equilibrium when these prevail. Markets generally tend towards the equilibrium. In the example above, market forces have determined that Q(e) of the good will be produced. In other words society, without taking any form of collective decision, will have allocated that amount of resources needed to produce Q(e) to the production of this good; no more and no less.

The free market will also solve the distribution problem. Figure 3.1 shows that if the good were zero-priced consumers would demand Q(3) of it. This is greater than Q(e), which means that at the equilibrium quantity (or the quantity associated with any positive price) there will not be enough of the good produced to satisfy everyone's want for it. Some form of rationing is necessary. In the free-market system, only those who are willing and able to pay at least P(e) get the good.

3.2.2. *Changing the given 'state of the world'*

The virtues of the free-market system come to light when the result of a change in the 'state of the world' is analysed. Suppose that the demand for jogging shoes rises for no other reason than that the goods suddenly become fashionable. If before the change in fashion demand was equal to supply, there will now be an excess of demand over supply. For the reasons just explained this will put pressure on prices to rise. As prices rise the good will become more profitable for the producers who, motivated by nothing more than their own self-interest, will increase production. New firms attracted by the profitability will enter the market. This means that scarce resources will be diverted from other things and into the production of jogging shoes. This will continue until a new equilibrium is reached. The unregulated free market will ensure that resources are diverted into the production of those things that society demonstrates it wants.

In the same way, discovery of a new more efficient production technique means that the same level of output can be produced at less cost. The resulting increase in profitability encourages self-interested producers to increase production of the good and new firms to be attracted into the industry. If demand was equal to supply before the change, there will now be an excess of supply over demand. This will put pressure on prices to fall, so consumers as well as producers will benefit from the new technology. The free market will have done its work.

Perhaps the most appealing aspect of the free-market model is that an ideal situation arises as a result of both consumers and producers acting entirely in their own interests. In particular, the principle of 'consumer sovereignty' applies; each individual is deemed to be the best judge of his or her own welfare and will spend a finite income in that way which maximizes his or her own well-being. The consumer rules. If informed people choose to smoke, drink, eat fatty foods with lots of salt, and take no exercise because this is how they maximize their own welfare, then any measures by government such as taxing, subsidizing, or restricting the production or availability of goods, is an abrogation of the principle of consumer sovereignty and by definition leads to a reduction in individuals' welfare. Since, again by definition, *social welfare* is the sum of the welfare of all the individuals in society, then social welfare is maximized when each individual is allowed to maximize his or her own welfare.

3.3. Why intervene in the free market? The case of cigarettes

Cigarettes are perhaps a less than ideal example to use to illustrate the arguments for government intervention because the analysis is partly unusual in the element of addiction. According to economic theory, a rational smoker will stop smoking without hesitation if the utility from smoking does not outweigh the costs. It is apparent that such rationality will not always apply in this case. Nevertheless, the example otherwise provides an unusually good illustration as will be shown. Given the topicality of the smoking debate, it is hoped that the reader will look beyond the unusual attribute in order to glean the main message from this example.

Placing a tax on a particular good is one way of intervening in a free market, and tobacco is one of the world's most highly taxed products. Virtually every country has been taxing tobacco since long before the health risks of smoking were known, mainly because tobacco duty is an easy way to collect tax and the demand for cigarettes does not vary greatly with its price. (For empirical estimates of the price elasticity of demand for cigarettes see Chapter 8.)

When the link between smoking and ill-health was established, governments further intervened, to varying degrees, in the market for cigarettes by such means as placing restrictions on who could buy them, limiting the number of places where they could be smoked, funding health education and other anti-smoking information, forcing manufacturers to put health warnings on cigarette packages, and severely restricting cigarette advertising. At the same time pressure groups against smoking have grown in strength and become ever more vociferous.

Together these suggest that there must be sound arguments for intervening in the freely made choice of smokers. Despite this there is a powerful pro-smoking lobby which clearly feels that such intervention is wrong. The principal argument of the pro-smoking lobby is that anyone who is willing to accept the risks associated with smoking should be free to do so. The first question to address is whether or not people are genuinely aware of the risks they face.

3.3.1. *Perfect information: the first assumption*

For market forces to work in the way outlined in Section 3.2.1, it is necessary for both producers and consumers to have perfect knowledge. If, for example, the realization that smoking is harmful to health causes consumers to alter their demand for cigarettes, then the original demand level which was based on ignorance, must have been sub-optimal.

Smoking has long been officially recognized as a hazard to health (Royal College of Physicians 1962, US Department of Health, Education, and Welfare 1964). It has been implicated in the increased incidence of lung cancer, coronary heart disease, bronchitis, emphysema, bladder cancer (Doll 1983), Crohn's disease (Tobin *et al.* 1987), and even excess facial hair in women who smoke (Hartz *et al.* 1987). Moreover, women who smoke during pregnancy increase the risk of having low birth-weight babies (Doll 1983), and of childhood cancer in their offspring (Stjernfeldt *et al.* 1986). Even those who do not smoke face increased risk of lung cancer (Wald *et al.* 1986) and of childhood respiratory illness (Chen, Li, and Yu 1986) if exposed to secondhand cigarette smoking.

Despite overwhelming evidence of the health risks of smoking and a great deal of publicity highlighting these risks, a survey conducted in the US 16 years after the famous Surgeon General's Report (US Department of Health, Education and Welfare 1964) found, as shown in Table 3.1, that 40 per cent of smokers and 25 per cent of non-smokers said that they did not believe that smoking reduced life expectancy. The reported difference between smokers' and non-smokers' perceptions is striking. For those who believed that smoking did reduce life expectancy, the difference in perceptions between smokers and non-smokers is repeated with 30 per cent of non-smokers, but only 17 per cent of smokers, believing that smoking reduced life expectancy by 6 years or more.

The same observations can be made for the UK population as shown in Table 3.2, although the differences between smokers' and non-smokers' perceptions are not as wide as in the US. Moreover, only about 10 per cent of smokers and 2 per cent of non-smokers did not believe that smoking could damage health.

It seems that the message may have been better received in the UK than in the US, but it must be emphasized that in all cases the data are based on *reported* perceptions. It is possible that smokers are reluctant to admit publicly their true perceptions or the reported differences may be due to better informed

Table 3.1 Estimated life expectancy loss from smoking by smoking status, United States, 1980

Estimated life expectancy loss from smoking (years)	Smokers (percentage)	Non-smokers (percentage)
0	40.9	24.7
less than 2	5.6	5.0
2–6	27.5	27.5
more than 6	16.9	29.7

Note: Percentages do not add to 100 due to omission of don't knows
Source: Roper Organization quoted in Ippolito and Ippolito 1984

people choosing not to smoke. Nevertheless, it would appear from Tables 3.1 and 3.2 that there remains some lack of awareness of the risks of smoking.

If it is accepted that some people smoke out of ignorance of risk, does this necessarily mean that the public provision of information is justified? After all, consumers make many 'wrong' decisions out of ignorance or lack of complete

Table 3.2 Perceived health damage from smoking by sex and status, Great Britain, 1982

	Smokers		Non-smokers	
	Heavy (percentage)	Light	Ex-smokers (percentage)	Never smoked
Males				
Can damage	72	69	82	88
Too much can damage	14	19	12	7
Cannot damage	10	9	3	2
Females				
Can damage	74	67	83	86
Too much can damage	12	21	10	9
Cannot damage	9	7	4	2

Source: Office of Population Censuses and Surveys 1984

information. They buy inappropriate cars, choose the wrong holidays, and pay high prices for inferior quality goods when better quality goods can be obtained elsewhere at lower prices. It is rarely argued that government has a duty to provide information to assist consumers in making welfare-maximizing choices in such circumstances. There are two principal reasons why cigarettes (and other hazardous or preventive goods) are different.

3.3.1.1. Information through experience   The first factor concerns the way in which consumers gain the relevant information through experience. While it is often impossible to judge accurately, prior to consumption, exactly how much utility a good will yield, consumers will usually realize after consuming the good that the utility derived was more than expected, or less, and will adjust future consumption accordingly. Consumers thus learn from experience how to maximize utility from their limited incomes.

Chapter 9 will explain how goods which increase the risk of future ill-health provide a type of negative utility from the knowledge that consumers may be doing themselves harm. Such knowledge, however, cannot be gained through experience—except after many years of exposure to the risk and after the damage is done. In the short- to medium-term, someone who is unaware of the hazardous attributes of cigarettes will not become aware by smoking. Total post-consumption utility cannot therefore be assessed in the case of hazardous goods.

3.3.1.2. Producer provision of information   The second factor concerns the way in which consumers gain information through advertising. The objective of advertising is to make consumers aware of the product's existence and virtues, and to increase demand. Advertising can and, because it is in the interest of the producers too, usually does provide the consumer with the information necessary to make informed choices and allow unregulated markets to operate efficiently. Producers will stress in their advertising whatever aspect of their product is most likely to increase sales. In the case of goods which promote health, such advertising is likely to address the health promoting attribute as well as the other attributes, such as good taste, fun to use, and so on. But in the case of hazardous goods, advertising is unlikely to stress the hazardous attributes of the good since this will have the opposite effect, i.e. it will decrease demand. Furthermore, warning information is more likely to be withheld when risks are long-term and the problem of attributing legal liability makes it difficult to sue the sellers of hazardous products. It is most unlikely that tobacco companies would have put health-warning messages on their product and in their advertising without government pressure backed by legislative power.

Unlike the market for normal goods, the unregulated market for cigarettes will not provide the information necessary to make informed choices, and consumers cannot gain such information from experience of consuming the good. There is thus a case for the public provision of information.

To justify other forms of government intervention such as taxing cigarettes, putting restrictions on their advertising, restricting their purchase, and prohibiting smoking in specified areas, requires a deeper analysis of the nature of this market. Before returning to the specific case of cigarettes, there is a general problem of risk awareness which should be mentioned.

3.3.2. Cognitive dissonance

There is considerable evidence to show that even when it is possible scientifically and objectively to determine levels of risk, people consistently under- or over-perceive them regardless of their *awareness* of the facts (Cohen 1981). One factor which is known to affect perception is the clustering of unwanted outcomes. For example, because road traffic fatalities tend to occur in ones and twos while air fatalities tend to occur as major disasters, the well publicized safety record in aviation relative to road travel is not reflected in the fears associated with the two modes of travel. Similarly, industries which have relatively low accident and death rates will be perceived as being dangerous places to work if those accidents and deaths that do occur tend to happen in headline-making catastrophes.

Perceptions are also affected by the degree to which risks are imposed or are accepted voluntarily. Governments recognize that people accept higher risk levels when freely chosen than when imposed (Mole 1976). There is an argument that when there are gross under- or over-perceptions of true risks, paternalism (i.e. professional 'objective' decision making) may help people to make more efficient choices. This may apply in the case of smoking.

3.3.3. No externalities: the second assumption

The description of the workings of the free market assumed that the utility yielded by a good goes to the consumer alone and that the costs of consumption are borne by the consumer alone. There are, however, instances when the consumer is not the sole recipient of the utility—positive or negative—and not the sole bearer of the costs. In these situations rational consumption decisions made by individuals may be socially sub-optimal since consumers will only consider costs and benefits to themselves. Individual decisions may leave society worse off, thus justifying some form of state intervention in the freely made choices of individuals. It is not difficult to demonstrate that in the case of cigarettes many costs and (dis)benefits are borne by non-smokers. First, external resource costs are examined.

3.3.3.1. *Health care costs*   Perhaps the most obvious external resource costs are those incurred in the treatment of illnesses caused by smoking. Rarely are full health care costs borne by the individuals who are ill. In the UK, where health care is zero-priced and funded from taxation, it has been estimated that the annual cost of smoking to the National Health Service is £370 million (House of Commons 1986.) In countries with essentially private health care systems the state still normally bears a large share of the total health care costs. The US, for example, has Medicare and Medicaid, and around 40 per cent of the total health care costs are paid by government. Most people who do not qualify for government assistance have some form of private insurance cover. This means that only rarely will the full health care costs of smoking be borne by the individuals who are ill. It has been estimated that the direct annual health care cost of smoking in the US is $8.2 billion (1976 prices) (Luce and Schweitzer 1978).

There is also increasing evidence that smoking can damage the health of others, either through what has become known as 'passive smoking' (Garfinkel *et al.* 1985) or via placental transfer in the case of a mother who smokes during pregnancy (Stjernfeldt *et al.* 1986). Clearly the health damage and health care costs to these individuals are entirely external.

3.3.3.2. Output lost through sickness absence Illnesses induced by smoking impose not only health care costs, but also costs in terms of the output lost because of sickness absence from work. The cost of such absence is the value of the reduction in output.

Not all such output receives financial reward. Housework, for example, produces something that is clearly of value. It is possible to estimate its value by various means, say by using the cost of employing a home-help as a proxy. Normally, though, the cost of lost unmarketed output will be borne by the ill individual or the family. If the family is taken to be the decision-making unit then there are no external costs involved.

With financially-rewarded output (i.e. when people are paid for the work they do) the cost of employing them is usually used as a proxy for the value of the output they produce. When such output is lost, it is often not the sick individual who bears the cost, because sickness benefit paid from social insurance has the effect of transferring the cost to a third party. The cost of sickness absence is thus largely external. In the UK, one estimate puts the cost of sickness absence caused by smoking at 50 million working days lost per year (Royal College of Physicians 1977) worth £2500 million at 1987 prices.

In addition to health care and lost output costs, there are a host of other sources of external resource costs which are difficult to quantify but which are known to exist. These include the cost of fires caused by smoking and the extra cleaning due to smoking.

3.3.3.3. External intangible costs There can be little doubt that smoking imposes considerable external costs of a less tangible kind, in addition to the external resource costs just discussed. Many non-smokers receive considerable disutility from other peoples' smoking, as witnessed by the increasing demands for, and provision of, non-smoking areas in public and private places.

Consumption by fully informed, rational consumers is based on a comparison of marginal utility and cost. The discussion above has shown that such smokers will not take into account a number of costs and benefits that, from a society-wide point of view, ought to be included. By acting in their own interests smokers will make socially sub-optimal decisions unless there is some mechanism acting on behalf of those adversely affected.

3.3.4. *No merit good qualities: the third assumption*

It has long been recognized in the literature that certain classes of goods are '. . . considered to be so "meritorious" that an amount over and above what is demanded through the free market by private buyers is provided by the state.' (Musgrave 1959). This suggests that some elite decides that consumption is below the social optimum. If the values of the elite are accepted then merit good qualities provide an argument for intervention.

This same line of reasoning has been applied to health care—and in theory could be applied to prevention—but has been couched in the more familiar externality terms. This argument states that yet another form of externality exists, based on the notion that some people are altruistically concerned about other peoples' consumption of certain 'meritorious' goods. Culyer (1976) has argued that, 'Individuals are affected by others' health status for the simple reason that *most of them care*' (p. 89 author's emphasis). If Culyer is right, and prevention is a merit good because man cares about the health of his fellow man, then another form of externality exists in addition to those discussed above. Those who care receive utility directly from others' consumption of health-promoting goods and negative utility from others' consumption of hazardous goods. In this sense, cigarettes can be viewed as de-merit goods. The existence of the humanitarian externality is not undisputed (see, for example, Sugden 1980), but if it is there, then the fully informed rational consumer will again not be taking everything that is relevant into account and will make socially sub-optimal choices.

3.3.5. *No public goods elements: the fourth assumption*

Free-market models assume two characteristics of all goods:

(1) rivalness: meaning that if one unit of a good is consumed by one individual that unit is no longer available to be consumed by another;
(2) excludability: where it is possible to prevent anyone who does not pay for the good from benefiting from its consumption.

When these two assumptions do not hold then the free-market model ceases to be an efficient allocator or distributor.

The draining of a malarial swamp is an example of a public good. The rivalness principle does not hold since the benefits of malaria eradication gained by some individuals do not mean that there are fewer benefits left for others. The excludability principle does not hold either, since those who do not pay for the drainage cannot be denied its benefits. Swamp drainage would thus not be provided by private firms operating in free markets.

The provision of information about the health damage caused by cigarettes is another example. Acquisition of the information by some individuals does not prevent others from acquiring it, and it would be difficult to exclude those who did not pay for it from acquiring it. Hence such information is generally provided as a public good.

3.3.6. *No supply side imperfections: the fifth assumption*

Sections 3.3.1 to 3.3.5 were all concerned with market imperfections on the demand side. There can be any number of imperfections on the supply side. The distinguishing feature of them all is that market forces are not able to perform as they would where firms compete to produce at lowest cost. In all cases, suppliers are able to behave in a way contrary to the laws of competition thus reducing or even eliminating the advantages of free-market operations.

For example, the free-market model predicts that an increase in demand will lead to a price rise. This in turn will cause an increase in output as producers shift resources to the production of the good whose demand has risen. The increase in total output of this good can happen either by:

(1) existing firms increasing output;
(2) new firms being attracted into the industry;
(3) some combination of the two.

More output will only be produced if there are no barriers to entry, i.e. anyone who wishes to go into production of this product is able to do so. If one firm had a monopoly on the production of a good it could react to an increase in demand by retaining the old level of production, increasing its prices, and increasing its profits. The free market will not work to the benefit of society as a whole in this case.

Even in competitive markets it is possible for firms to collude and engage in all manner of unfair trading practices. Generally, the more an industry is concentrated in the hands of a few relatively large firms the greater is the potential for unfair practices. Since many industries are characterized by 'increasing returns to scale', (a situation where unit costs fall as output is expanded), concentration is often inevitable. The tobacco industry is a classic example.

The history of that industry is one of monopoly power on both sides of the Atlantic. In the early years of the twentieth century, James 'Buck' Duke's American Tobacco Company (ATC) had a virtual monopoly on cigarette production in the US. Fear of an attempt by Duke to take over the UK industry led thirteen British tobacco companies to merge, in 1901, to form the Imperial Tobacco Company. Rather than compete with each other, ATC and Imperial joined forces to form British American Tobacco (BAT), with Duke as its first chairman. The US Supreme Court eventually deemed the ATC monopoly in America to be against the public interest and ordered it to be dismantled. At the same time ATC sold most of their holdings in BAT to British investors, leaving BAT the world's biggest tobacco multinational (Taylor 1984).

Despite such attempts to encourage competition, the tobacco industry is today still concentrated in the hands of a few multinationals and state monopolies. Five giant multinationals (BAT, Philip Morris, R.J. Reynolds, Rothmans International, and American Brands) share 35 per cent of world cigarette output, with a further 55 per cent produced by state monopolies. This leaves only 10 per cent of world production in the hands of private companies, and even here dominance is by a few large firms (Tucker 1982). The free-market model's assumption of perfect competition is clearly not applicable in the market for cigarettes. That is one reason why the profitability of tobacco multinationals tends to be higher than that of companies in other industries (Booth, Hardman, and Hartley 1986).

3.4. Discussion

The main message from this chapter is that the case for no government intervention in the market place appears to be justified only in the case of perfect markets. Once market imperfections exist on either the demand side or the supply side, then the virtues of the free-market model are weakened. Imperfections do not, of course, mean that society *will* be in a sub-optimal situation in terms of social welfare—the existence of a benevolent monopolist, for example, is a possibility—but the greater the imperfections, the greater the potential for sub-optimal situations, and the stronger is the case for some form of intervention.

The above analysis suggests that economics may have a lot to offer in the evaluation of the extent to which various prevention activities lead to or inhibit the maximization of social welfare. It is to the role of economic appraisal that we now turn.

4 Economic appraisal in prevention

4.1. The role of economic appraisal in prevention

The emphasis of Chapter 1 was on the notion that since resources will never be sufficient to satisfy all human wants and desires, choices have to be made. There are many ways to choose how to allocate resources, and everything from historical precedent to a system of allocating resources to those with the most political power has at least some advocates. Economics does not claim to offer the only criteria for choice. Rather, economic appraisal is advocated as an aid to decision making and never as a substitute for it.

The main criterion for choice used in economic appraisal is economic efficiency, or trying to maximize the benefits from available resources. Since putting society's resources to one use means doing without the benefits that could have been obtained by using the resources in some other way, maximizing benefits means minimizing opportunity costs.

Economic appraisal in the area of prevention can help to do this by addressing such questions as:

1. Could more morbidity and mortality be avoided by rearranging the way that prevention resources are currently deployed?
2. If more resources were made available for prevention, which way of using them would achieve the maximum reduction in morbidity and mortality?
3. If a given decrease in morbidity and mortality were to be achieved, which way of achieving it would entail the minimum opportunity cost?

Another type of question addresses the worthwhileness of transferring resources into prevention from other uses:

4. Do the benefits of devoting more resources to prevention outweigh the opportunity costs?
5. If the answer to the above is yes, how many more resources should be devoted to prevention?

Questions of the type 1–3 are tackled through the use of *cost-effectiveness analysis* (CEA) or *cost–utility analysis* (CUA), where the available budget is fixed and the maximum benefits are sought, or the objective is fixed and the minimum cost method of achieving it is sought. Questions like 4 and 5 are tackled by *cost–benefit analysis* (CBA), where both the budget and the objective (or the extent to which the objective could be met) are variable. In CBA the costs and the benefits are expressed in comparable units—money values. This helps with decisions on whether and to what extent to pursue a policy or programme. In CEA the benefits are generally in measurable units of effectiveness, such as years of life gained, or reductions in the number of cigarettes smoked, while in CUA they are in terms of quality-adjusted life-years (QALYs) gained. These two types of appraisal address the question of how most efficiently to pursue a programme or policy, *given* that the decision to pursue it has already been taken.

In addition to the preventive actions carried out by individuals, prevention is undertaken by a host of different organizations, government departments, voluntary agencies, and charities, as well as through the more formal health care sectors. Hence, questions such as 1 above require a great deal of information and are particularly difficult to answer.

If cost–benefit and cost-effectiveness appraisals were costless in terms of time as well as resources, then most decisions concerning the use of prevention resources would be subject to thorough economic appraisal so that all choices could be made with full knowledge of all relevant costs and benefits. Clearly, appraisals are not costless and the number of choices is so vast that it would be unrealistic to suggest that all be subject to formal appraisal. However, as was pointed out in Chapter 1, economics is a way of thinking as well as a set of techniques.

It is within this way of thinking that a framework for planning the use of prevention resources and a framework for appraising programmes can be found. In both cases it is the way that problems are considered that is of importance, not the formal application of a prescribed set of rules. After discussion of these frameworks this chapter will return to the formal techniques of appraisal mentioned above.

4.2. Programme budgeting: a framework for planning in prevention

While specific prevention initiatives may be directed at specific preventable conditions, all share the common broad objective of reducing future morbidity and mortality. Any attempt to devise an overall prevention strategy should begin by looking at the way in which resources devoted to prevention are currently being deployed and applying questions of types 1 to 3 above. This is not to suggest that reducing mortality by preventing coronary heart disease cannot be valued differently from similar reductions in mortality by preventing road traffic accidents. Indeed priorities will be an inevitable part of a broad prevention strategy. Nevertheless, the 'broad brush' approach does keep the notion of a common objective at the forefront.

At this level, planning is in terms of client or disease groups rather than specific initiatives and requires information that matches the nature of the questions asked when broad priorities are considered. For example, the question 'Should more be done to reduce smoking prevalence?' requires different information from that needed to decide whether or not a specific anti-smoking campaign should be run. In the latter case the decision will ideally be based on a full awareness of the costs and benefits of the proposed campaign.

On the other hand, the decision to give priority to anti-smoking generally implies that expenditure on anti-smoking should be increased as a proportion of total expenditure on prevention. This requires some knowledge of what percentage of total prevention expenditure is currently going to anti-smoking efforts and some means of monitoring whether this percentage increases over time as planned. The problem is that some anti-smoking activity is carried out by doctors, some by voluntary agencies, some by health education bodies, some by employers, and so forth, and the total from all of these is normally not available to provide the overall picture.

Programme budgeting seeks to break down a total 'budget'—in this case a total prevention initiative—over a number of 'programme' headings. While programme budgeting allows inputs (costs) to be related to activity measures (which may be used as proxies for outputs), it does not attempt to relate costs to final outputs (in terms of reduced morbidity and mortality) and is thus not evaluative. It can, however, indicate areas where evaluation may be called for.

Programme budgeting depicts the current deployment of resources across broadly-defined programmes, showing current allocations to different groups and hence to different objectives, in addition to relating these expenditures to indicators of output. Past trends in programme growth indicate how the programmes developed and give an opportunity for monitoring and checking whether what was intended is occurring. Finally, programme budgeting can assist with planning by allowing various potential scenarios to be presented, indicating possible policies that might be pursued within and between programmes (Mooney, Russell, and Weir 1986).

Since the programme budgets must sum to 100 per cent of the total budget, the concept of opportunity cost is clear. With programme budgeting, an argument that greater priority must be given to programme X emphasizes that there must also be a relative loser. The expected gains in benefit from expanding programme X must now be viewed in terms of what sacrifice this entails in the losing programme. It also focuses attention on *marginal* programme changes, which are the basis of the framework for the evaluation which follows. For example, an increase in the anti-smoking programme from say 5 per cent to 7 per cent of total prevention expenditure represents some marginal increase in expenditure. The expected benefits resulting from this marginal increase in cost can be weighed against the marginal loss of benefits associated with an equal cost reduction in one or some combination of the other programmes, to help ensure that the most efficient use of the overall budget occurs. Examples of prevention programme budgets are given in Chapter 10.

4.3. Marginal analysis: a framework for appraisal

The programme budgeting approach, and the example of anti-smoking *versus* immunization, highlight the idea that most decisions concern marginal changes in existing programmes. The questions of whether we should screen more often or whether more people should be included in a screening regime are more typical than whether there should be screening for the disease—yes or no? Full blown cost–benefit and cost-effectiveness analyses cannot be undertaken on all resource allocation choices, but a framework which is firmly grounded in the cost benefit approach can be helpful even when the full appraisal techniques cannot be used.

Marginal analysis is based on the principle that resources are scarce. It explicitly recognizes that all potentially preventable morbidity and mortality will never be prevented, and refutes the indefensible argument that human life and suffering are priceless and prevention is therefore beyond consideration of cost. Opportunity costs do not cease to exist simply because one refuses to recognize them!

An interesting feature of marginal analysis is that by focusing on the margins of programmes it ignores *total* costs and benefits, as well as total need; neither of which is relevant to the question of whether a programme should be expanded or contracted. For example, in the case of cervical cancer screening the question of whether or not to provide screening is no longer an issue in many industrialized nations. Whether more should be done in this area, say by screening more often or including younger women in the screening regime, is being debated. If this is the issue, then all that is required is an awareness of the *extra* costs of expanding the programme and the *extra* benefits which will result.

Marginal analysis emphasizes that these extra (marginal) costs and benefits are likely to vary as programmes are expanded or contracted, in a predictable manner. In the case of cervical cancer screening, the *first* women who will be included in a rationally applied screening regime will be those at highest risk. (Strictly, it should be those for whom there is potentially the greatest benefit, presuming the costs of screening per woman are constant across all risk groups.) As the programme is expanded, progressively lower and lower risk women will be included. For example, the programme might first recall women after 10 years. If more resources were available, this might be reduced to 8 years, 5 years, or 3 years. It would, of course, be possible to include all women every month in the regime, but as the likelihood of detecting any pre-cancerous lesions among women screened less than a year before is small, few would advocate including them in screening programmes. Thus the benefit per screen of screening every 10 years (in terms of pre-cancerous lesions detected) is likely to be higher than that of screening every 8 years which will in turn be higher than that of screening every 5 years, and so on.

In the same way, screening a given population once may miss some pre-symptomatic cases (false negatives). If the population is screened twice to double-check, and assuming the time delay between screens is not so great that many new cases develop, the number of cases picked up on the second screen will be much lower than on the first, similarly for the third; and so on. Thus the marginal benefit falls as the programme expands as shown in Figure 4.1.

At the same time it is normally the case that as a programme is expanded *marginal costs* arise. For example, setting up a screening clinic in a city centre may attract 60 per cent of eligible women. To increase the uptake rate to 80 per cent may require mobile clinics to reach women in remote areas who will not come to the city centre clinic, thus increasing the marginal cost. To reach 90 per cent may also involve an advertising campaign—again at extra cost— and to reach 100 per cent, assuming it were possible, might mean sending nurses out to women's homes to undertake domiciliary screening. Marginal cost curves of such programmes normally look like CC in Figure 4.2.

How can this help with the sorts of questions in Section 4.1? To avoid (temporarily) the problem of placing a monetary value on the benefit of detecting a case of pre-symptomatic cancer, two sub-programmes which have benefits in the same measurable units of effectiveness—in this case pre-

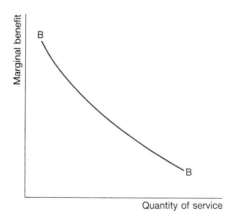

Fig. 4.1 Diminishing marginal benefit.

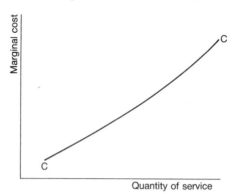

Fig. 4.2   Rising marginal cost.

symptomatic cases detected—will be compared. The cost and benefit figures might look as in Table 4.1.

If £400 000 were available to spend on detecting pre-symptomatic breast cancer, and all were spent on sub-programme A, the total number of detected cases would be 505. Spending all on B would detect 78 cases. Attempting various combinations costing a total of £400 000 will show that more benefits are possible than by spending the whole budget on either sub-programme alone. Four units of A and two of B will yield 560 detected cases, a total which cannot be exceeded by any other combination while keeping within the budget constraint.

It will be noted that, at these levels, the ratio of marginal benefit to marginal cost in each programme is the same. It can easily be shown that at any combination where these ratios are not the same, reducing spending on the

Table 4.1   Hypothetical costs and benefits of screening for breast cancer

	Sub-programme A				Sub-programme B			
Units	Marginal cost £000	Total cost £000	Marginal benefit	Total benefit	Marginal cost £000	Total cost £000	Marginal benefit	Total benefit
1	200	200	400	400	90	90	60	60
2	20	220	40	440	20	110	10	70
3	30	250	30	470	40	150	5	75
4	40	290	20	490	50	200	2	77
5	50	340	10	500	60	260	1	78
6	60	400	5	505	65	325	0	78
7	70	470	0	505	75	400	0	78

sub-programme where the ratio is lower and using the released resources to expand the other, will produce a greater total benefit at no increase in total cost.

In practice it will not always be possible to determine accurate costs and benefits in this way, but it is the principle that matters. Viewing the information in this way, focusing on estimates of marginal costs and benefits, ignoring total costs and benefits, and ignoring total need, constitutes a framework that can help in the pursuit of efficiency even when accurate and detailed information is not available.

4.4. Cost–benefit analysis

Questions of types 4 and 5 (see Section 4.1 above) are addressed by cost–benefit analysis which is based on the principle that every programme—or any change in the level of any programme—involves the use of resources which could have been put to other purposes. There is thus always a sacrifice involved, and the decision rule of CBA is to pursue only those policies where the value of the benefits they generate is at least as great as the value of the sacrifice required to bring them about. When two or more policies are competing for the same resources, then that with the greatest excess of benefit over cost is to be preferred. The justification for the approach is that it points out those ways in which social welfare can be increased. CBA emphasizes the need to be explicit about the exact nature of the problem, the objectives, and the policy options. This crucial first step of carefully identifying the study question has not always been properly applied. As Sugden and Williams (1978) have said:

The designer of a poorly thought-out cost–benefit study may believe that it will answer questions that it logically cannot. Worse, he may believe, after the study is complete, that it *has* answered them—in which case public decision-making may actually be made less rational by the use (or misuse) of his analysis. (p. 231)

4.4.1. *Costs and benefits*

The key feature of both costs and benefits is *value*. In principle, a benefit is anything which someone would be willing to pay something for, and a cost is anything which someone would be willing to pay something to avoid. Whether or not payment is actually made is of no consequence to its value.

Ideally, CBA will include all costs regardless of who bears them and all benefits regardless to whom they accrue, on the principle that if net benefit is positive it is possible to redistribute some of the gains from the beneficiaries to compensate completely the losers and still leave society better off. Thus programmes pass or fail the cost–benefit test according to whether they could make *society* better or worse off. A different viewpoint could be used. This could, for example, be that of a profit maximizer, but adoption of the societal viewpoint is one of the key features of CBA that distinguishes it from a mere financial appraisal, and it ensures that decisions will be taken in full awareness of all the implications of the decision.

Examples of different types of costs and benefits are given in Table 4.2. The important feature to note is that *it does not matter whether costs and benefits*:

(1) have market prices attached;
(2) are tangible or intangible in their nature;
(3) are borne by individuals, families, or by public or private institutions.

It is worth pointing out to those who (mistakenly) believe that economics is about money, that there are certain financial transactions which appear to be costs or benefits, but which are neither. Such *transfer payments* can be identified by the fact that they do not make society as a whole any better or worse off. Sickness benefit is an example.

When an individual cannot work because of illness or injury, a cost is incurred in that the output which would have been produced is lost. Society is worse off in that Gross National Product is lower than it would otherwise be.

Table 4.2   Some examples of costs and benefits of prevention

Costs:
    Tangible
        professional's time
        drugs and equipment
        leisure time used in consuming prevention
    Intangible
        increased inequity in health of population
        pain associated with vaccination

Benefits:
    Tangible
        resource savings
        increased productivity
        more leisure time
    Intangible
        avoided pain
        longer life
        reduced anxiety

The value of the loss is normally estimated by the price that the individual's output would have sold at (which is also the gross cost of employing that individual for the time involved, if markets are functioning perfectly).

If the individual concerned happens to receive sickness benefit to compensate him or her for the lost earnings, then at least some of the burden is *transferred* from the sick individual to the employer or the state. The movement of money from the latter to the former is a transfer payment not a cost. If sickness benefit were to be included among the costs (since it is a cost to the paying agency) it would involve double counting. If it were to be included among the benefits (since it is a benefit to the recipient) it would have the effect of negating a true cost. Thus transfer payments have no place in CBA— although their distributional effects may be important, as will be explained shortly.

4.4.2. *Positive cost or negative benefit?*

The above has indicated what should and what should not be included among the costs and benefits in CBA. The problem still remains of which is a cost and which a benefit. In fact when analysing individual programmes on their own, it makes no difference whether something is called a positive cost or a negative benefit. Adding 5 kg to the left side of a balance scale has an identical effect to removing 5 kg from the right. A programme that passes the cost–benefit test cannot be made to fail by calling some positive costs negative benefits or *vice versa*.

But whether something is called a positive cost or a negative benefit does matter when different programmes are being compared in terms of cost–benefit *ratios* if there is inconsistency in the way cost and benefit elements are expressed in two analyses. This problem is easily avoided by expressing the result in terms of *net benefits* where the nomenclature used cannot affect the final figure.

$$\text{Net benefit} = \text{total benefit} - \text{total cost}$$

(But see below for an important refinement.)

4.4.3. *Valuing costs and benefits*

Having identified and measured all costs and benefits the next step is to weigh one side against the other and this requires some common unit of measurement. Since all costs and all benefits are *valued*, and since a monetary symbol is used to express values, money is normally used as this common measure (although in principle anything would do). It is worth emphasizing that the £ or $ represents an expression of value rather than a sum of cash.

When market prices are available they are often accepted and are broadly acceptable as unambiguous indicators of the value of costs or benefits. Thus if the price of an ounce of gold is ten times that of an ounce of silver, the implication is that the value of gold is ten times that of silver. If there is doubt about whether market prices truly reflect value, then adjustments can and should be made.

When market prices are not available, it is still often possible to tease out values. For example, although housework is normally unpaid labour, society clearly puts a positive value on it. Any programme which prevents the loss of housework by preventing illness or injury should include this among its benefits. Indirect ways can often be found to tease out its value. In this case the cost of employing a home-help to do this work could be used as a proxy.

Anything up to and including the value of reducing the risk of death can be estimated, at least crudely, by various means. The value of fewer road deaths, for example, can be teased out by asking people how much they are willing to pay to reduce, by some small amount, the risk of dying in a motor accident (Jones-Lee, Hammerton, and Philips 1985).

4.4.4. *Dealing with uncertainty*

The above raises a general problem with measuring and valuing costs and benefits. For one thing it is not possible to obtain perfectly accurate information on every variable in the analysis and for another the future is inevitably uncertain. The need to make assumptions is therefore inescapable.

Suppose for example that a screening programme will run for 10 years and use a detection machine and 1600 hours of nurse time per year valued at £X per hour—the gross cost of employing a nurse for an hour. A cost–benefit analysis might assume that the same amount of time, the same real cost of labour, and the same yield in terms of cases detected, will apply to each year of the programme. Clearly, without any reason to suspect otherwise this would be a wholly realistic assumption. It may, however, turn out that after the programme failed the cost–benefit test and was given the red light not to proceed, an improved machine was developed that increased the number of cases detected per 1000 hours of screening time. Would this matter? Would the programme have passed the cost–benefit test if the improved machine had been available at the time and the appropriate figure for the cost per case detected was included? More generally, are the results of the appraisal *sensitive* to changes in the assumptions?

Sensitivity analysis is a refinement of CBA that essentially repeats the appraisal using different assumptions. If the probabilities of assumptions being right or wrong are incorporated, it can be made analogous to statistical confidence limits which do not change the conclusion, but do show decision makers how confident they can be in the results. Even without knowing the probabilities, sensitivity analysis can show which assumptions most undermine confidence in the conclusion. When results are shown to be highly sensitive to particular assumptions, further investigation and refinement of those assumptions can be valuable.

4.4.5. *Dealing with time*

Dealing with time is crucial to the appraisal of prevention since nearly all prevention seeks to avoid future illness and injury. Within the formal health care sector, resource expenditures on prevention programmes mean forgoing the benefits of health which could have been realized through curative treatments. In the case of individuals engaging in prevention, again the cost— in terms of whatever is the nature of the opportunity cost—is incurred today in order to realize future benefits.

As individuals and as a society we are not indifferent as to when costs are incurred and when benefits are realized. If all else were equal, we would prefer to delay costs as long as possible and receive benefits as soon as possible. It is easy to show how the *value* of any cost or benefit changes according to when it occurs.

Imagine you have been fined £100 for exceeding the speed limit in your car, but are given a choice; pay now, or pay in a year's time. For simplicity assume there is no inflation. (We could just as easily say you would have to pay £100 adjusted for inflation in a year's time.)

You quickly realize that since banks pay interest on deposits, you could deposit some amount less than £100 today that would grow to £100 in a year's time. If the bank pays 5 per cent interest on deposits (or with inflation, if its *real* rate of interest is 5 per cent) you would find that £95.24 will earn £4.76 interest over the year giving you £100 when you came to close your account. The choice facing you today is between paying £100 to the court or putting £95.24 into the bank.

If the choice were between paying today or paying in 2 years' time, you would find that at 5 per cent interest a deposit of £90.70, if left alone, will grow to £100 in 2 years' time. In this case your choice today is between paying £100 to the court or putting £90.70 into the bank. The actual amount you eventually pay is the same in all cases, but clearly the farther into the future it occurs, the lower is its 'present value'.

Economics uses *discounting* to express all future costs and benefits in terms of their 'present values'. In the example, the future fine was discounted at a rate determined by bank interest rates. In more complex cases the choice of discount rate is not so straightforward. The rate used to discount future costs and benefits for social programmes will not necessarily reflect the personal discount rate of any individual. The higher an individual values present costs and benefits over future ones, the greater will be that individual's personal *time preference rate*, and the more highly he or she will discount the future when making individual choices.

The principle of discounting future costs and benefits is not a disputed issue, but the choice of the appropriate rate of discount is. When the time lag between the incurring of costs and the realization of benefits is long, the results of a CBA can be sensitive to the choice of discount rate and a sensitivity analysis varying the discount rate may be appropriate.

The *present values* of the costs and benefits are worked out by the formula:

$$\left[PV = \frac{A}{(1+r)^n} \right]$$

where A = the nominal amount (in this case £100)
       r = the rate of discount
      n = the number of years from now when it arises

4.4.6. *Implied values*

As many people find the placing of monetary values on health benefits to be at best distasteful it must be emphasized that the issue at hand is whether such valuations should be explicit or implicit, not whether or not they should be made. They *are* made every time a decision to pursue, or not to pursue, a particular course of action is taken.

The cost–benefit balance could be worked out based only on those cost and benefit elements that are readily and uncontentiously expressed in money terms, leaving out such intangibles as life-years gained. If the value of benefits exceeds the value of costs then the programme is clearly worth pursuing since the addition of the value of these life-years can only reinforce the conclusion already reached.

Often, without considering intangibles, the costs will outweigh the benefits. In this case a conclusion cannot be reached concerning whether or not the programme passes the cost–benefit test since not all costs and benefits have been considered (see quote by Sugden and Williams, Section 4.4).

However, a decision will be taken with or without economic appraisal on whether or not to pursue the programme. Anyone arguing in favour of the programme is implicitly valuing the intangibles at *at least* the amount by which the costs exceed the benefits, since this is the cost of the life-years gained. Anyone arguing against the programme is implicitly valuing the life-years gained at less than this amount. Valuations of intangibles such as increases in life expectancy and relief of suffering cannot be avoided. They are implicit in every decision which is taken. The only real choice is whether the valuation is made explicit or left implicit. CBA can be of much help to decision makers if it is remembered that the cost–benefit approach is not advocated as a substitute for other methods of decision making.

(CBA) does not seek to replace the sound or educated judgment of the decision maker. . .
It is the principal aim of all evaluative research, and CBA is certainly no exception, to
provide a more considered and sound information base for policy decision. (Knapp
1984, p. 116)

4.5. Cost-effectiveness analysis

Most of the principles of CBA are also relevant to the other types of appraisal
which fall within the cost–benefit framework. Cost-effectiveness analysis
(CEA) differs from CBA in that benefits are expressed in units of effectiveness,
but are not valued (explicitly). This difference has radical implications.

First, without valuing output it is not possible to show how the benefits of
one programme compare with those from programmes with different outputs.
It is thus not possible to say whether benefits exceed opportunity costs, which
in turn means that it is not possible to say whether and to what extent a
programme should be implemented. Put more simply, CEA cannot question
the objectives of the programme, but must take them as given. It cannot
address questions 4 and 5 (Section 4.1) and it cannot deal with programmes
that have multiple outputs (objectives). For example, CEA cannot compare a
cholesterol reduction programme whose only output is in terms of reduced
coronary heart disease with an anti-smoking programme that reduces
coronary heart disease as well as lung cancer, bronchitis, and emphysema—
except if the output is constrained to a single dimension such as lives saved.

Second, on the assumption that an objective will be pursued, CEA recognizes
that there are normally alternative ways of pursuing it. This type of appraisal
can show which alternative will produce the greatest benefit for a given
expenditure or which alternative will achieve a given benefit at least cost. It
addresses type 1, 2, and 3 questions (see Section 4.1).

From the above it is evident that cost-effectiveness is a relative state and CEA
can only identify the most cost-effective of the alternatives. There will always
be a winner and that winner will not necessarily pass the cost–benefit test. It is
therefore wrong to state, as is so often done, that something *is* cost-effective.
Something can only be *more* or *less* cost-effective than something else.

Although it can only answer a more limited set of questions, CEA avoids the
difficult step of monetary valuation. It can also be simpler in that the analysis
need not consider anything that does not affect the ranking of the alternatives.
If, for example, in a breast cancer screening programme, different combinations of mammography, thermography, and physical examination are
compared, the costs incurred by women in travelling to the clinic can be
ignored. They will be identical for all of the alternatives and cannot affect the
ranking. In CBA they ought to be included.

The other principles discussed in Section 4.4 still apply. The social welfare approach is still preferred, discounting is still relevant, transfer payments are not (except for distributional reasons), the principles of looking on the margin still apply, and so on.

4.6. Cost–utility analysis

While any measure of effectiveness can be used in CEA, there is one measure that has received particular attention. This is years of life gained. Since the gain of a life-year in pain and immobility will not be valued as highly as a healthy life-year, non-monetary weights are attached to this output to reflect quality. The result is the 'quality-adjusted life-year' (QALY) and the technique of appraisal that compares programmes in terms of this weighted unit of output is *cost–utility analysis* (CUA).

Many prevention and treatment programmes have this common output despite the very different illnesses or injuries with which they are concerned. When they are compared in CUA, that with the lowest cost per QALY is relatively the most efficient, and is the one which should be expanded first.

Because of the weighting of life-years, CUA can arguably lie somewhere between CBA and CEA. However, since QALYs are not valued in monetary units they cannot be weighed against opportunity costs to answer the 'whether' or 'how much' questions that CBA addresses. CUA is therefore better seen as a variant of CEA.

4.7. Clarifying social goals

CEA and CUA are concerned with *technical efficiency*. They are about how to achieve a given objective as efficiently as possible. CBA is concerned with *social efficiency*. It seeks to maximize the benefits obtainable from limited resources. If maximizing net benefits was the only social objective then CBA would be the only decision technique needed. This is clearly not the case; efficiency is only one criterion for choice.

As well as the amount of net benefit, society will also be concerned with the way that benefit is distributed. The term *social welfare* can be used when social efficiency is broadened to take on board additional criteria such as *equity*.

It is helpful to distinguish between equity and equality. Equality is about equal shares, equity is about fair shares. An equal distribution of prevention would have everyone consuming the same amount. An equitable distribution would have individuals consuming prevention according to some fairness rule, for example, in proportion to the risks they face (their *need* for prevention).

Allocation in free markets, however, is determined by demand based on a willingness and ability to pay, and willingness and ability to pay are not necessarily related to need. If need is defined in accordance with some notion of social equity, then it can be argued that the free-market solution to distribution is fundamentally inequitable. It can further be argued that appraising prevention by the efficiency criterion alone will be insufficient, as the most efficient solution may be inequitable.

There is no agreed best way of dealing with equity in economic appraisals. At one extreme is the view that economists should deal with efficiency and leave distributional issues to others. After all, if the fundamental problem concerns the distribution of income and wealth, then it is up to the distributional branch of government to sort things out. As Culyer (1976) so succinctly puts it 'In short, if the poor have too little money, give them the cash'.

A more commonly held view is that efficiency and equity are inextricably linked. While an efficiency based CBA is by no means value-free, one difficulty in trying to integrate efficiency with equity is that, because there is normally a trade-off between the two, value judgements become more prominent in determining the best course of action.

As most economists prefer to reduce the risk of imposing their own values on social decisions, economic appraisals normally follow one of two paths. The first examines the efficiency consequences of applying different equity criteria, but leaves decision makers to judge whether the equity gains of less efficient alternatives outweigh the efficiency losses. The second attempts to build value judgements into the appraisal by teasing out some form of consensus values. For example, if it can be ascertained that the benefits of detecting pre-symptomatic illness in people from lower socio-economic groups are valued more highly than those from higher socio-economic groups, then distributive weights could be assigned to benefits according to who receives them. The CBA decision rule will thus incorporate a 'fairness test' directly into the appraisal.

This approach forces decision makers to consider distributive consequences explicitly and systematically. From a theoretical point of view, this is preferable, but in practice decision makers may find this more difficult than the first method.

Efficiency is not the only basis on which to determine a social goal of worth. An alternative egalitarian approach will be more concerned with distribution than with totals. If a 'fairness test' is applied in addition to the cost–benefit test, then CBA (with other criteria) can be said to be concerned with *social welfare*.

4.8. Conclusion

The theory of economic appraisal is inherently attractive. At the same time it has to be remembered that it cannot be value-free and that it is never advocated as a substitute for decision making. Criticism of economic appraisal more often concerns the way it is used in practice than the theoretical aspects. In the two chapters which follow examples of economic appraisals in prevention are reviewed. Methodological issues arising, and models of good practice are discussed in Chapter 7.

5 Case studies in primary prevention

5.1. Introduction

It is easy to agree with the principles of economic appraisal while at the same time doubting its practicality. The idea of weighing gains against sacrifices is pleasing in theory, but is it really possible to put a money value on reduced pain and suffering? Is there any point in applying the principles of economic appraisal when the aetiology of a disease is largely unknown or subject to controversy?

This chapter and the two which follow show that these problems are by no means insurmountable. This chapter and Chapter 6 review economic appraisals in primary and secondary prevention respectively, focusing on specific preventive measures, how they were appraised, and the results. Chapter 7 concentrates on methodological issues and practical problems encountered in these studies, highlights how they were tackled, and the lessons to be learned.

The studies reviewed in Chapters 5 and 6 were selected to cover a wide range of topics. Other criteria for selection were the soundness of the approach and the potential impact of the results. It is clearly impossible to provide a comprehensive review of all the issues involved in the application of economic appraisal to prevention, but the studies discussed do show some of the breadth of issues already tackled, thereby revealing the diversity of policy issues in this field and providing evidence on the efficiency, or otherwise, of various preventive initiatives. In addition, they reflect the current state-of-the-art of economic appraisal in prevention.

The studies of secondary prevention are necessarily concerned with preventive services provided by health professionals. It is worth noting, though, that of the ten primary prevention topics listed below, only two— immunization and family planning—are provided exclusively by health professionals. The other eight involve a host of agencies which are not part of the formal health care sector. The selected topics covered in Chapter 5 are:

—immunization
—family planning
—health education about diet

—food regulation
—fluoridation
—health education about smoking
—tobacco taxation
—road safety
—environmental health
—occupational health

5.1.1. *Definition of terms*

Economic appraisal considers all costs, regardless of who bears them, and all benefits regardless to whom they accrue. As indicated in Table 4.2, costs and benefits are classified as either tangible or intangible, according to whether or not they are readily measurable. Thus the time of nurses used in any programme is a tangible cost since it can measured, or at least estimated, to the nearest minute. The saving of nurse time is a tangible benefit for the same reason. Anxiety is an intangible cost. While its presence or absence may be noted, it is very difficult to measure the degree of anxiety in any objective or reliable way. For the same reason reduced pain is an intangible benefit. Because tangible costs and benefits are measurable, they tend to be given careful consideration in most economic appraisals. However, as will be shown, and perhaps understandably, the equally important 'intangibles' sometimes receive far less rigorous treatment.

For the purposes of these chapters, costs and benefits are further classified as priced or unpriced, according to whether there are associated market prices. Thus while an hour of nurse time is priced, since nurses are paid a market wage, an hour of a voluntary worker's time is unpriced. This distinction has no bearing on whether or not either is a cost (or its saving is a benefit). If using either of these resources in a prevention programme means that something else has to be forgone—because that resource would otherwise have been used to produce benefits elsewhere—then a cost is incurred. Similarly increased productivity due to better health is a benefit regardless of whether or not those whose health is improved get paid for that increased productivity. Society does not pay for housework, but it values it. Other terms such as 'non-economic' or 'non-financial' which are often used in studies such as these, are eschewed in these chapters because they are unclear and often inaccurate.

5.2. Some examples of economic appraisal in primary prevention

5.2.1. *Immunization*

Immunization can be extremely effective in preventing disease, and may ultimately eradicate a disease, as happened with smallpox. Immunization is also of particular interest in economics in that it not only confers benefits on those immunized, but also confers important external benefits by reducing the risk of transmission to non-immune people.

In this section we review two economic appraisals of immunization programmes. The first looks at the costs and benefits of a programme that at the time of the study had been running for over 20 years. It thus questioned a long established strategy. The second compares different immunization strategies for preventing one disease.

5.2.1.1. *Tuberculosis* The past contribution of immunization to the decline in mortality and morbidity in industrialized countries is difficult to assess. McKeown (1979), for example, has argued that better nutrition, hygiene, sanitation, and family planning have had a much greater impact than vaccination or any other medical interventions. Figure 5.1 provides some evidence to support his contention. The graph also suggests that the elimination of BCG vaccination (to prevent tuberculosis) is unlikely to result in a rise to the disease levels experienced earlier. This raises the general point that as the incidence of certain diseases declines it may be necessary to question whether existing immunization policies, which may have represented efficient

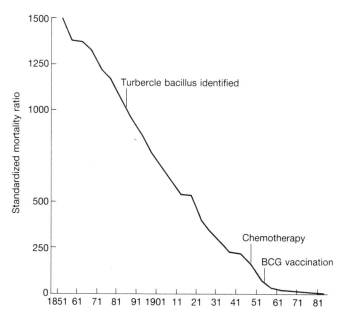

Fig. 5.1 Standardized mortality rates for tuberculosis, both sexes combined, 1851–1985 (1950–1952 = 100), England and Wales.
Source: Swerdlow 1987

uses of resources when first initiated, remain efficient with the lower prevalence. Stilwell (1976) addressed this very issue.

Stilwell examined the resource consequences (tangible, priced costs and benefits) of BCG vaccination against tuberculosis for English schoolchildren. Five out of every six schoolchildren in England were given a BCG injection at around 13 years of age. The other either refused, had immunity already, or had medical contra-indications. BCG gives 80 per cent immunity for 15 years (Medical Research Council 1972).

The British Thoracic and Tuberculosis Association (1975) had calculated that 100 000 inoculations in 1975 would prevent 12 cases of tuberculosis in 1975, 10 in 1976, and fewer in each succeeding year. The cost per inoculation to the health service was £0.99. Thus, 100 000 inoculations would cost £99 000. The projected savings were calculated as the reduction in treatment costs for the cases of tuberculosis prevented, and reduced time off work in the future. The average savings per case ranged from £400 without hospitalization to £1370 with 87 per cent of cases hospitalized, this being the proportion of all cases requiring hospitalization at that time. The total savings would be worth between £40 000 and £70 000 leaving a deficit of at least £29 000. Moreover, in the future, the proportion of cases hospitalized was expected to decline, making treatment cheaper, and the effectiveness of BCG (the number of cases prevented by 100 000 inoculations) to fall. Hence the ratio of cost to saving was expected to increase to at least 7:1 by 1985. Even under the assumption that each estimate had been wrong by 25 per cent in the direction that would bias the results against BCG, the ratio would still be at least 4:1 by 1985. Other countries have acted on such evidence (Conway 1990).

There are of course the intangible and unpriced consequences to be taken into account, such as the pain or discomfort of the injections and of TB, and parents' or others' unpaid time spent caring for those with TB. On the other hand, using health service resources for something other than BCG might alleviate even more illness, distress, and discomfort, in total.

Stilwell suggested that a better programme would be to select for immunization those at high risk—for example, immigrants from countries where tuberculosis is more prevalent, and contacts of notified cases. A selective programme would almost certainly give much greater net benefits. The position in the UK in 1991, however, is that the Health Departments still recommend BCG for all school children at 13 years of age.

5.2.1.2. *Rubella*   The second study reviewed here is concerned with a situaation where serious ill-health in an unborn child is avoided by the prevention of a relatively trivial disease in a pregnant woman. Rubella is a disease where harmful effects in infected people are rare, but which can cause heart defects, deafness, blindness, and mental retardation in around 30 per cent of the children of women who are infected in the first 3 months of pregnancy.

There are several possible strategies to deal with this problem. In one, complete eradication of the disease is sought by mass immunization of the whole population. In another, only schoolgirls are vaccinated, since only female immunization is required to avoid the possibility of infecting fetuses. Schoenbaum *et al.* (1976) conducted a cost–benefit study of the immunization strategy against rubella that had been adopted in the USA—immunizing both girls and boys at around 2 years of age—and compared this with other strategies such as that in the UK where until recently only girls were immunized at around 12 years of age.

Their study question—'Which strategy would produce the greatest net saving of resources?'—meant that parallel cost–benefit analyses were conducted for each strategy. Clearly, by focusing solely on resource savings, these studies were incomplete.

Schoenbaum *et al.* were able to show that combining rubella immunization with measles immunization would produce a greater excess of benefit over cost than giving it alone. Given a choice between immunizing 2-year-old girls and boys and immunizing 12-year-old girls, the latter strategy would produce a greater net benefit and also be more effective in reducing congenital rubella syndrome. Combining both, so that girls would be inoculated twice, would provide a smaller net benefit than the previous strategy by around $20 million, or $20 per girl.

These net benefits included only the tangible, priced resource consequences. Unpriced benefits, such as the avoidance of parents' unpaid time devoted to caring for a disabled child, and unpriced costs such as the time spent taking children to be immunized, were omitted. The intangible benefits of avoided distress to both children and parents if disability is prevented, and intangible costs such as the pain of the injection were also left out.

The information on effectiveness was not based on a randomized controlled trial, and many assumptions and estimates had to be made about the consequences of different policies for rubella prevention. Owing to the uncertainties introduced by this, and the exclusion of unpriced and intangible effects, the reliability of the conclusion that immunizing only 12-year-old girls seems to be the most efficient strategy, is not certain. It should, however, make policy makers at least devote careful consideration to abandoning such a policy. It is unclear to what extent this information influenced the decision by the UK Health Departments to include rubella immunization as a part of a new triple vaccine (measles, mumps, and rubella) offered to all infants since 1990.

5.2.2. *Family planning*

McKeown (1979), among others, has argued that family planning has been a major factor in improving the health of the populations of industrialized countries. While some contraception may provide other benefits, such as the prevention of sexually transmitted diseases, in this section we consider only the prevention of unwanted pregnancies.

Birth control methods differ in both their effectiveness and their cost. Trussell (1974) has analysed a wide range of methods in terms of their relative cost-effectiveness. Included were the condom, spermicides, oral contraceptives, intra-uterine devices (IUD), the diaphragm, vasectomy, abortion, and certain combinations of these. All are available under the NHS in the UK.

The costs of some methods are repeated over time as their use is continual (e.g. condoms) while for others, such as vasectomy, the cost is incurred only once. Trussell constructed a profile of the costs over a period of 15 years, and discounted future costs using a 10 per cent rate of discount. The costs of each method are given in Table 5.1.

The effectiveness of the different methods was compared in terms of 'use effectiveness'. This allows for failure of the method itself, inadvertent misuse of the method, and occasional deliberate risk-taking. Allowance was also made for an observed 18.3 per cent spontaneous abortion rate, and periods of non-exposure to the risk of pregnancy, i.e. during pregnancy and one month after birth.

The effectiveness of each method is the difference between the actual number of pregnancies or births, and the expected number if no method of birth control were used. The use effectiveness of each method is also shown in Table 5.1.

Of the methods incurring expense, vasectomy is the most cost-effective. Coitus interruptus which is costless in terms of the clinic's resources, could be combined with abortion thus preventing all the unintended births that would arise from using this method, and at around £1 000 might be described as efficient. The costs in Table 5.1 do not, however, allow for such intangible factors as the use-utility of the method, by which criterion coitus interruptus might well score less highly than vasectomy. It also ignores the ethical and highly emotive aspects of abortion, especially when it is considered as a method of birth control.

Table 5.1 shows vasectomy to be more cost-effective than such methods as oral contraceptives, diaphragms, and spermicides. It can, of course, be argued that given the permanent nature of vasectomy it is misleading to compare it with methods which can be stopped if a planned pregnancy is desired. Nevertheless, Trussell's findings are still useful. There were around 3000 vasectomies performed in England in 1983, on men whose average NHS waiting time was about 4 months—making a total wait for all these men of about 1000 years. If the NHS was meanwhile providing these men and/or their partners with alternative forms of contraception, then Trussell's evidence indicates that there would be fewer unintended pregnancies and lower resource costs through cutting these waiting times.

Table 5.1   Costs and effectiveness of family planning methods

	Clinic costs, £ per 100 users over 15 years at 10 per cent discount rate	Use effectiveness per 100 women per year		
		Pregnancies	Pregnancies prevented	Births prevented
'Chance'	0	50	0	0
Abortion	3089	64	−14	52
Coitus interruptus	0	20	30	25
Condom	3068	17	33	27
Diaphragm	2944	16	34	28
IUD	1616	6	44	36
Oral contraceptives	3492	14	36	29
Rhythm	0	31	19	16
Spermicide	5116	24	26	22
Spermicide + condom	6794	5	45	36
Vasectomy	1122	0	50	41
Condom distribution*	1730	17	33	27
Spermicide distribution*	3778	24	26	22

* Without medical supervision or other clinic services
Source: Trussell 1974

5.2.3. *Health education about diet*

Diet is argued to be a major contributor to modern Western mortality patterns. It is claimed to contain too much saturated fat, increasing the risk of coronary heart disease; too much salt, increasing the risk of hypertension (high blood pressure) and leading to heart and cerebrovascular disease (stroke); too much sugar, leading to tooth decay and contributing to obesity; and too little fibre, increasing the risk of cancer of the colon. There have, however, been major shifts in public attitudes to foods in the 1970s and 1980s, including a substantial switch of consumption from butter to margarine and from white bread to wholemeal. Just how the message about healthy eating has reached consumers is less clear.

    Goss (1985) examined the costs and benefits of a potential public education campaign in Australia to inform people of the health hazards of high consumption of salt and to persuade them to halve their salt intake, which at that time was between 10 and 40 times in excess of minimum requirements. Around 25 per cent of deaths in the age group 35–64 years were said to be linked with hypertension, and the proportion of a population with hypertension to vary directly with sodium intake. A 50 per cent reduction in salt consumption would bring most Australians into the range 40–100 mmol sodium intake per day. Other calculations suggested that such a reduction in sodium intake would prevent blood pressure increasing with age. It was estimated that this would save 432 000 lives over a 40-year period from 1991 to 2031, equivalent to 6 345 000 life-years saved.

Goss suggested that the government could achieve a 50 per cent reduction in salt intake by a thorough and extensive mass health education campaign advising people to avoid adding salt in cooking or at the table, to switch to low salt margarine or butter and low sodium bread, and to eat less of highly salted foods. In addition, he considered that there would be a need for follow-up studies of hypertension prevalence, and further surveys of foods to check sodium content and nutritional labelling. On the basis that A\$260 million was spent on food and alcohol advertising in Australia in 1984, Goss reckoned that the maximum cost of a health education campaign would be A\$300 million over the first 5 years and A\$3 million per year over the following 40 years (1985 prices).

Using the above estimates (and a 5 per cent rate of discount) the cost per life-year saved would be A\$208. This cost is low in comparison with other methods of dealing with hypertension. For example, an earlier study by Stason and Weinstein (1977) had calculated the costs and effects of screening for and treating high blood pressure in the USA. When converted to 1985 Australian dollars, their estimates of the cost per (quality-adjusted) life-year gained through the drug treatment of people with moderate to severe hypertension (diastolic blood pressure over 105 mmHg) were A\$9520 assuming full compliance and A\$20 620 with lack of adherence to medication.

Goss undertook sensitivity analyses of his results to show the effect of more pessimistic assumptions. He found that even if the benefits of sodium reduction had been over-estimated by a factor of ten, and if only half the population reduced their sodium intake by 50 per cent the cost per life-year saved was still only A\$4160.

Goss's calculations were speculative, but tests of sensitivity to changes in the important parameters provided strong indicative evidence that salt reduction would save more life-years at lower cost than screening and administering anti-hypertensive drugs. A more recent review of the international evidence has confirmed that reducing salt consumption would indeed be likely to have major beneficial effects on mortality rates (Law *et al.* 1991).

5.2.4. *Food regulation*

Sometimes governments wish to go further than just educating people about the health hazards or benefits of consuming certain foods and decide to regulate the types, or standards, of foods available for consumption. In this section we review two studies, both concerning the prevention of salmonellosis, but via different channels of transmission.

5.2.4.1. *Non-pasteurized milk* In 1980, the UK government deferred a decision to ban the sale of non-pasteurized milk in Scotland pending studies of the costs and benefits of such a ban. The proposed legislation was confined to Scotland since the consumption of non-pasteurized milk and consequent milk-borne infections, were considerably higher there than in other parts of the UK.

One of the present authors undertook such a study (Cohen *et al.* 1983). The main benefits of the proposed ban would be in reductions in milk-borne salmonellosis and *Campylobacter* enteritis, milk-borne tuberculosis and brucellosis no longer being a problem in the UK. The study focused solely on salmonellosis for two reasons. First, the evidence on incidence of *Campylobacter* enteritis was patchy. Second, as will be shown below, the proposed ban was almost certain to pass the cost–benefit test even with only a partial examination of benefits.

This study was more comprehensive than those reviewed above as it was not confined to health service and non-health service costs, but also included other priced and unpriced resource consequences of *Salmonella* infection. These are shown in the upper part of Table 5.2. In addition, the study considered minimum estimates of the value of two types of intangible costs—pain, grief, and suffering, and loss of life. These were based on figures then used by the Department of Transport (Morgan and Davies 1981) to decide on how much should be spent on road improvement projects. It was estimated that the annual cost of milk-borne salmonellosis in Scotland was £93 000. This figure was used as the minimum value of the benefits that the ban would confer.

The costs of the ban were dependent on the way in which the farmers who supplied non-pasteurized milk would react. If they had their milk pasteurized by the Milk Marketing Board, the costs would be negligible as the Board's tankers passed by almost every farm anyway and the marginal cost of heat treating the extra milk was estimated to be close to zero. If they decided to pasteurize on the farm, then the cost of equipment, heat treatment, and maintenance would work out at about £2300 per farmer per year. Thus if more than 40 farmers decided to take the latter course, the cost of the ban would exceed the minimum estimate of the benefits. A survey of producer-retailers virtually ruled out this possibility.

It is worth noting that any loss of utility to consumers who genuinely prefer non-pasteurized milk ought to be included among the intangible costs of the ban. This possible cost element was ignored in this study because earlier changes from non-pasteurized to pasteurized milk went undetected by consumers. It was only later, when the labels were changed to indicate that the milk which they had been drinking for months was pasteurized, that complaints were received!

Table 5.2 Costs of an outbreak of milk-borne salmonellosis, £

Tangible costs	
Direct	
All medical	33 738
All laboratory	3629
Veterinary	910
Environmental health surveillance	6075
Indirect	
Visitors travel to hospital	2873
Lost output (paid employment)	36 864
Lost output (housework)*	9222
Lost leisure time*	240
Total tangible costs:	93 551
Intangible costs	
Pain, grief and suffering*	33 450
Loss of life*	109 000
Total intangible costs:	142 450
Total cost of the outbreak	236 001
Number of reported cases	654
Cost per case	361

Source: Cohen *et al.* 1983
*=minimum estimates

The conclusion from this study was that on best estimates the benefits of the ban would outweigh the costs. The study was thus influential in the decision taken by the government, in 1983, to proceed with the ban.

5.2.4.2. Poultry In Scotland, poultry has always been responsible for many more cases of food-borne salmonellosis than milk. In the mid-1980s the UK government was contemplating the irradiation of poultry (Advisory Committee on Novel and Irradiated Foods 1986) as a means of killing *Salmonella* and other bacteria. The costs and benefits of such a measure were assessed by Yule *et al.* (1986).

The authors estimated that the total cost of reported cases of poultry-borne salmonellosis in Scotland was at least £200 000 per year. Unlike milk-borne salmonellosis, however, which tends to occur in well-reported outbreaks, poultry-borne salmonellosis often occurs as isolated cases that are usually unreported. One study (Roberts 1985) estimated that less than 5 per cent of total cases may be reported. On the assumption that for every reported case there were twenty unreported, and that unreported cases caused no mortality or hospitalization but incurred roughly 30 per cent of the other costs of the reported cases, the cost for unreported cases in Scotland would be at least £980 000 per year. The total minimum estimate of the benefits of irradiating all poultry consumed in Scotland was thus £1 180 000. As with the study by Cohen *et al.*, this estimate was a minimum because of the exclusion of other benefits of irradiation such as reductions in other pathogens and the increased shelf-life of food.

The authors estimated the total costs (capital plus running costs) of irradiating all poultry to be approximately £910 000 per year—clearly lower than the minimum estimate of the benefits. Scotland would be better off by requiring the irradiation of poultry.

This result, however, was sensitive to the assumptions made; particularly that concerning unreported cases. If there were only ten unreported cases for every reported case, or if unreported cases cost only 10 per cent of reported, then the benefits would be less than the cost of irradiation. On the other hand if much higher values were placed on the reduction of pain, grief, suffering, and death, then this would again raise the benefits over the costs.

The potentially crucial intangible cost of public concern over irradiation was not considered in this study. Popular belief that food irradiation is dangerous has probably delayed its implementation. The value put on this concern is likely to be the ultimate decisive factor. This study is helpful in that it shows the magnitude such a value must have if food irradiation is to be rejected on cost–benefit grounds.

5.2.5. Fluoridation

The fluoridation of drinking water as a way of protecting the population, particularly children, from dental caries is another measure that has strong emotive elements attached to it. It has been extensively researched from the economic perspective.

Fidler (1977) compared the dental records of 3 025 young people who lived in two adjacent areas in the south of England. In the first area, fluoride (1 ppm) had been added to the water supply since 1956. The second area had unfluoridated water. There was a sizeable difference in the amount of treatment received by each group, with a saving of around £1.50 per person for those in their teenage years who lived in the fluoride area. Although not based on a randomized controlled trial, Fidler's samples were matched for age and social class. As all the children used the same dentists there is little reason to attribute these results to anything other than fluoride.

The costs to the fluoridated area had previously been estimated at £0.06 per person (Borough of Watford 1969, quoted in Davies 1973), or about £0.40 per child. Even after discounting to take into account the delay between the 'investment' in fluoridation and the 'return' in terms of savings in dental expenditure, there is still a strong indication that fluoridation saved more than it cost in terms of tangible, priced, resource consequences. The intangible benefits to children of avoided tooth decay and toothache, and fewer missing and filled teeth can only strengthen the conclusion that investment in fluoridation was worthwhile.

These results for the UK have been corroborated by a number of studies in other countries. In the US, Nelson and Swint (1976) estimated that fluoridating the water supply of Houston, Texas, would produce a 'social profit' (present value of resource savings minus resource costs) of $1.103 million (1975 prices). In Australia, Doessel (1980) did a similar exercise for Townsville. He used extensive sensitivity analyses to test the robustness of the conclusion, and found that the benefits exceeded the costs under all but the most unrealistic assumptions.

More recently, however, there has been a questioning of the need for water fluoridation because of the reduction in dental caries which has occurred since sales of fluoride toothpaste rose in the 1970s (c.f. Figure 5.1). Jackson (1987) has discussed these views, but concludes that given current costs of water fluoridation and of dental treatment, fluoridation would only need to prevent decay in three teeth per person before the age of 15 to pay for itself. Unfortunately, Jackson did not apply discounting. If he had (using 5 per cent) then he would have shown the need for only two prevented caries per person in the first 15 years to justify the fluoridation on (limited) cost–benefit criteria. Despite the widespread use of fluoride toothpaste, water fluoridation still appears to be a profitable investment.

5.2.6. *Health education about smoking*

There are many possible ways of measuring the effectiveness of health education campaigns, ranging from knowledge gains, through attitude changes, and ultimately behaviour change—that is, a change in the demand for a preventive or hazardous good. It is, ideally, only the last which should be considered as the true measure of success. Unfortunately, in the case of tobacco it is notoriously difficult to estimate the effect of health education on demand. An evaluation of anti-smoking advice in terms of overall costs and benefits would need to estimate the reduction in smoking brought about by the campaign. Despite evidence of quit rates for campaigns aimed at specific groups of people who have demonstrated a desire to quit, the success rates for campaigns aimed at wider audiences is largely unknown.

Recently, Williams (1987) appraised a campaign in which British general practitioners would give 5 minutes of anti-smoking advice to every male smoker over 40 who attended for consultation. He estimated the cost per quality-adjusted life-year (QALY) gained to be £167. This compares favourably with other medical interventions which have been evaluated in terms of cost per QALY gained (Gudex 1986), but is dependent on Williams' estimate of a 5 per cent quit rate being correct. There is some evidence concerning quit rates achieved by general practitioners giving advice to all smoking patients. For example, Russell *et al* (1979) observed a quit rate of 3.3 per cent. Considerably more evidence on both initial quit rates and relapse rates is needed before estimates such as those by Williams can be accepted with confidence.

On a smaller scale, there have been recent studies of the cost-effectiveness of some specific smoking cessation aids. These have tended to switch emphasis from education about the harm of smoking to helping people to overcome the addictive aspects of smoking, and helping to motivate people who have already expressed a desire to quit. Altman *et al.* (1987) have reported the costs and effectiveness of three smoking cessation programmes: a self-help quit smoking kit; a smoking cessation contest with prizes; and a smoking cessation class. These were part of a wider project to prevent illness known as the Stanford Five City Project.

The quit rates achieved were 21 per cent for the kit, 22 per cent for the contest and 35 per cent for the class. The marginal costs per quitter were $45, $61, and $266, respectively. Sensitivity analysis around these results was undertaken and indicated that only if the effectiveness of the kit were to drop to a 5 per cent quit rate would it cease being the most cost-effective option. The clear implication of this study was that given a limited budget, a sufficient number of interested smokers, and an objective of maximizing the number of quitters, then spending the budget on the self-help kits would achieve the maximum smoking cessation.

5.2.7. *Tobacco taxation*

Taxation is an obvious alternative to health education in the drive to reduce smoking. Unlike health education campaigns which consume tangible resources, increasing the tax on cigarettes does not. It could thus be argued that taxation is 'costless'.

It is most unlikely that any smoker would agree with such a view. From the smoker's point of view the increase in tax is not costless since he or she must pay more. Chapter 4 explained how tax revenue is neither a cost nor a benefit, but is a 'transfer'. The money which the smoker pays is identical to the revenue received by the exchequer, leaving society as a whole no better or worse off, aside from the administrative costs—which are a true resource cost, but are relatively insignificant in this case. From the social welfare point of view the tax is not a cost. However, there is another cost to the smoker which is not compensated from the perspective of society.

Economic theory states that the amount of extra utility that a consumer obtains from any good falls as consumption increases. Thus a smoker who has no cigarettes will get a great deal of utility from the first cigarette, a little less from the second, and so on. According to the theory, our consumer will demand cigarettes up to the point where the (falling) marginal value equals the (constant) price. There will be no consumption beyond this point since the value to the consumer of any additional cigarettes will be less than the cost. However, since the value of all but the last units purchased is greater than the price, the consumer receives what is called *consumer's surplus* on all units consumed (bar the last). Any increase in tax reduces the amount of consumer surplus, and this is the cost (loss of welfare) of taxation. Townsend (1987) looked at the cost of a rise in the price of cigarettes in the UK in terms of this welfare loss.

Townsend estimated how much consumers would lose if the UK government were to increase cigarette prices by raising taxes. First, she calculated demand curves for five different social classes (professionals, managers, skilled manual workers, semi-skilled, and unskilled). These curves showed the responsiveness of consumption to the change in price of a packet of cigarettes. Hence she estimated the approximate utility cost of the price rise. Consumers in social classes 2 to 5 would suffer a utility cost of between £1.00 and £1.40 per week owing to a price rise of £0.50 per packet (1980 prices).

Townsend estimated that smokers in social class 5 (unskilled manual workers) would reduce their smoking by around 30 cigarettes per week in response to a £0.50 price rise. If such consumers were aged 35 and each gained a year in life expectancy (the life-year accruing 35 years later), then the utility cost of the life-year gained would be about £2370 undiscounted. At a 5 per cent discount rate there would be a gain of 0.19 discounted life-years at a discounted cost of about £1160, giving a cost per life-year gained of £6100, which is not cheap!

Although these last calculations are speculative, they do illustrate that a price rise is not costless and, indeed, may be a more costly way of gaining life-years than providing education, advice, and assistance to help smokers quit, as outlined in the previous section.

Such calculations assume that smokers make rational choices about their consumption of cigarettes, which is unlikely given the addiction involved. They also assume no other benefits from reduced smoking-related morbidity and mortality. Since the evidence indicates otherwise, these results should be regarded as illustrative.

5.2.8. *Road safety*

In this section we review studies which address four preventive measures aimed at reducing road fatalities and injuries: alcohol regulation, motorcycle helmet laws, seat belt legislation, and speed restrictions.

5.2.8.1. *Alcohol regulation* Death on the roads is one of the many problems caused by alcohol which are of concern to public health policy makers. In the US particular disquiet has been expressed over the deaths of young people in alcohol-related road fatalities. Motor vehicle accidents are the leading cause of death among those aged under 35 and it is believed that alcohol is implicated in the majority of fatal accidents.

One initiative has been the passing of the Federal law on uniform minimum drinking age which penalizes those states that have a drinking age limit of less than 21. Saffer and Grossman (1986a, 1986b) compared the effectiveness of that initiative with a policy of raising the tax on beer which is the main alcoholic drink consumed by young people.

Saffer and Grossman looked at the period 1975–1981 during which 15 of the 48 contiguous states (i.e. excluding Alaska and Hawaii) had raised the minimum drinking age and during which the real price of beer had fallen. Statistics showed that motor vehicle death rates varied between states each year, probably owing in part to drinking age limit differences, and also varied over time for each state, probably owing in part to increased beer consumption during the period. As it would be unrealistic to attribute variations in the mortality rate to these two factors alone, Saffer and Grossman had first to isolate the effect of these factors from all the other influences on motor vehicle accident mortality rates during this period.

They controlled for other likely influences on drinking and driving by including additional explanatory variables in their statistical model. Their model provided a good explanation of variation in the mortality rate, in that about two-thirds of its variation was accounted for by changes in the included variables and was statistically significant overall.

The main results of the study were expressed in terms of the responsiveness of the mortality rate to changes in the beer tax and legal drinking age. They indicated that a 160 per cent increase in the tax on beer (approximately $2.40 (1986 prices) for a case of twenty-four 12 ounce cans) would decrease the motor vehicle accident mortality rate amongst youths aged 18 to 20 by 30 per cent. An increase in the legal drinking age from 18 to 21 would have the same effect. But would these two measures be equally efficient?

Since effectiveness is the same in both cases, the more cost-effective option is that with the lower cost. Neither tax increases nor age restrictions, however, involve costs in the usual sense of the term. Rather, the costs are in terms of losses in consumer's surplus (welfare) as in Section 5.2.7, on tobacco taxation.

Saffer and Grossman did not address this issue directly, but their analysis does provide the first step towards estimating the utility loss from both measures.

Clearly, if youths gained some consumer's surplus from continuing to consume some beer under the tax increase, but gained none by consuming no beer under the increase in the legal drinking age, then the tax increase would involve the smaller utility loss. This suggests that raising the beer tax could be more cost-effective than raising the legal drinking age, if the tax rise could be targetted at this age group alone.

5.2.8.2. Motorcycle helmet laws   In 1976, the US ended the imposition of financial penalties against states not having motorcycle helmet laws. Over the following few years over half repealed these laws. Muller (1980) estimated the costs and benefits of laws making the wearing of motorcycle helmets mandatory, basing his study on the accident experience of motorcyclists in Colorado, Oklahoma, and South Dakota, before and after these states repealed their helmet laws. The study included only the tangible priced resource consequences.

Muller reported that a safe motorcycle crash helmet could be purchased for approximately $30 (1979 prices) and would last at least 4 years. The reduction in helmet use from 94 per cent in the pre-repeal year to 43 per cent in the post-repeal year was thus estimated to have saved at most $0.47 million per 100 000 motorcyclists.

The total number of accidents did not change during this period, but there was a change in the distribution of injuries among motorcyclists involved in crashes with an increase in the proportion of major injuries. The extra medical care expenses from this change were calculated to be $1.1 million per 100 000 motorcyclists (1979 prices). Thus the net cost of repealing the helmet laws was $0.64 million per 100 000 motorcyclists, or around $16 million for all the states that repealed their helmet laws.

Muller's study did not consider the intangible cost of loss of freedom to choose whether or not to wear a helmet, nor the cost in terms of discomfort. At the same time, it also excluded the health benefits of reduced death, physical and mental disability and injury, as well as the benefits of extra output in employment. The freedom to choose not to wear a helmet would appear to have been bought at a high price.

5.2.8.3. Seat belts   One alternative to making the wearing of seat belts compulsory is to compel car manufacturers to install 'passive' seat belts (i.e. a shoulder belt attached to the car door in such a way that when the door is closed the belt automatically acts as a restraint). The costs and benefits of such a move were examined by Arnould and Grabowski (1981).

The cost of fitting passive belts was estimated to be between $25 (Volkswagen Rabbit) and $50 (General Motors Chevette). On the basis of a 10-

year car life, this represents an annual discounted cost per car of between $3.08 and $6.17. The total cost of supplying such belts on all 102 million cars in the US would thus be between $314 million and $629 million.

Experience with drivers of the Volkswagen Rabbit (who may not be typical drivers) showed that seat belt use was 33 per cent for those who had manual seat belts compared with 78 per cent for those with passive belts. As a result of greater usage, the fatality rate in accidents involving Volkswagen Rabbits with passive belts was half that for the same car with manual belts. Of course, seat belt use also reduces non-fatal injuries, and it was estimated that the total difference in medical care expenses between manual seat belts (assuming 20 per cent use) and passive seatbelts (assuming 70 per cent use) for both fatal and non-fatal injuries would be $180 million in total, or roughly $1.77 per car. This is less than the cost of installing the passive belt. Are passive belts therefore inefficient?

An earlier study by Thaler and Rosen (1976) had estimated the amount of money people were apparently prepared to pay to reduce their mortality risks. Using these estimates, Arnould and Grabowski argued that motorists should be willing to pay $300 to reduce the risk of fatality by 1 in 1000. If this figure were applied to the fatalities avoided by the fitting of passive seat belts, then the benefits would be increased to $8280 million in total or $81 per car. This would clearly outweight the cost of fitting passive seat belts.

It would be cheaper and more effective for the US to make the wearing of manual seat belts (currently fitted to all cars) mandatory. This, however, would be at the cost of lost freedom of choice. As with the motorcycle helmet laws discussed above, the Arnould and Grabowski study helps to quantify the price of this freedom.

5.2.8.4. *Speed restrictions* In an effort to conserve fuel, the maximum speed on US roads was reduced to 55 mph, in 1974. Though the fuel crisis came to an end, the speed restriction did not. This was largely due to an awareness that the lower limit was having a marked effect on road traffic injuries and fatalities. Forester, McNown, and Singell (1984) examined the costs and benefits of the 55 mph legislation.

Overall, the speed reduction was estimated to have saved 7466 lives per year although, interestingly, this was probably due more to a reduction in the variation in speeds between cars than to a reduction in average speed. The important of reducing the variation in speeds has been subsequently confirmed by Lave (1985), suggesting that the imposition of minimum speed limits near to maximum speed limits may be more efficient than reducing maximum limits alone.

Since the average age of those killed was 33.5 years, the 7466 road deaths prevented by the 55 mph limit would have produced an increase in total life expectancy of 316 000 life-years. At the same time, reducing speeds increases journey times. The 55 mph limit meant that an extra 456 000 life years were spent travelling.

Judgement concerning whether or not the speed limit produced net benefits for society, depends, therefore, on the value of life *versus* the value of time. On the basis of best estimates of values of life and time from previous studies, this study showed the speed limit to pass the cost–benefit test. However, this conclusion was far from robust.

5.2.9. *Environmental health*

Economists have been involved in helping to estimate the epidemiological relationship between pollution and health for many years. This has been no easy task for several reasons. First, there is the problem of determining what sorts of ill-health are caused by exposure to pollutants and establishing the extent of these causal relationships. Second, there is the difficulty of measuring the 'doses' of pollutants that people have received, since exposure varies by location, time of day, and season. People do not tend to stay in one location long enough to allow accurate long-term exposure to be measured. Joyce, Grossman, and Goldman (1986) overcame the latter problem by examining the effect of air pollution on neonatal mortality (deaths of infants less than 28 days old). Since it is unlikely that infants of this age will have moved location, the likelihood of measurement error is reduced.

Joyce *et al.* examined the effects of carbon monoxide, lead, sulphur dioxide, nitrogen dioxide, and total suspended particles on neonatal mortality across the 677 counties of the US with a population of over 50 000. Their analysis controlled for such other influences on neonatal mortality as use rates of family planning devices by teenage women, abortion rates, use rates of prenatal care, use rates of neonatal intensive care, cigarette smoking, and the proportion of women in higher risk ages for giving birth. Their main analysis concentrated on sulphur dioxide as this alone had a consistently negative and statistically significant effect. Separate analyses were done for the black and white populations. The results suggested that a 10 per cent reduction in sulphur dioxide levels would reduce the neonatal mortality rate by 0.4 per cent for whites and 0.5 per cent for blacks.

This study was particularly interesting in that, while the authors could not say what the overall costs and benefits of achieving a 10 per cent reduction in sulphur dioxide levels would be, they were able to identify how much society should be prepared to pay to achieve this reduction, given its willingness to pay for equal reductions in neonatal mortality by other means. For example, it was shown that a 2.6 per cent increase in the use of neonatal intensive care by whites, and a 5.3 per cent increase in use by blacks, achieves the same decline in mortality for each group at a total cost of $1090 million. Thus, they estimated that the benefits in terms of reduced neonatal mortality from a 10 per cent decrease in sulphur dioxide levels should be worth at least $1090 million. If such a reduction could be achieved at a cost of less than $1090 then a programme to reduce sulphur dioxide levels would be an efficient use of resources.

In their study, Joyce *et al.* used mortality rates of populations rather than data for individuals. Use of data that pertains to particular individuals may be potentially more reliable, particularly if comparative effects of more than one pollutant are being examined. This was the case with Portney and Mullahy (1986) who attempted to estimate the effects of pollution *and* smoking on health, when it was known that pollution affects the health of smokers and non-smokers differently.

Portney and Mullahy looked at individuals in city and suburban areas to determine the effects of different levels of ozone (average daily maximum 1-hour exposure) on respiratory-related morbidity. (Ozone is the principal constituent of smog.) After controlling for other influences, they concluded that the number of days of respiratory-related illness was significantly associated with the level of ozone. It was estimated that a 10 per cent reduction in the ozone level would reduce respiratory morbidity (measured as the number of restricted activity days) by 4.42 days per thousand individuals per 2-week period, or 12.64 million days per year for the whole urban adult population of the US.

A previous study by Loehman *et al.* (1979) had estimated the sums that individuals would be willing to pay for improved respiratory health. On this basis the value of reduced morbidity due to a 10 per cent reduction in ozone levels would be between $29 million and $139 million in aggregate. Portney and Mullahy did not attempt to estimate the cost of such an anti-pollution programme, but their estimate of its benefits could be used when estimates of the cost are made.

In both studies discussed in this section, the identified benefits were in terms only of reduced mortality or morbidity. The other benefits of reduced pollution, such as reduced damage to flora and fauna, increased agricultural output, or the aesthetic benefits of cleaner air, imply that the values derived in these studies are minimum estimates of the overall benefits.

5.2.10. *Occupational health*

The workplace may be a potentially efficient location for mounting preventive programmes to reduce risks that are not related to specific occupational hazards. Certain occupational groups, however, do face specific risks that are directly related to the nature of their work. There appear to be few examples of studies concerned with the costs and benefits of preventive measures to reduce specific occupation-related risks. This may be due in part to the measures being too specific to be of general interest, or because they are negotiated between employers and employees as part of general conditions of employment without detailing costs and benefits. Alternatively, they may be implemented without explicit consideration of their efficiency at all.

One of the few examples to be found in this area, and one which examined a classic case of a response to public and political pressure which had given no consideration to the issue of efficiency, is the study by one of the present authors (Cohen 1982). Following some well publicized outbreaks of hepatitis and smallpox among laboratory workers, the 'Howie Code'—the code of practice for the prevention of infection in clinical laboratories and post-mortem rooms (Department of Health and Social Security 1978)—was produced.

The Howie Code specified stringent safety standards, often involving large amounts of building renovation and the installation of expensive equipment. It was suspected that the cost of bringing clinical laboratories and post-mortem rooms to Howie standards would not be commensurate with the risks involved.

Cohen's study did not attempt to measure the cost of laboratory-acquired infection (whose reduction would be the benefit of the Code), but aimed to put the risks into perspective. While these risks were clearly greater than zero, the pattern of sickness absence among clinical laboratory workers was shown to be similar to that of the general working population and considerably lower than that of many major employers such as the Post Office or London Transport, which are not regarded as particularly dangerous organizations to work for.

The costs of the Code were also put into perspective by demonstrating that the cost of bringing just the two clinical laboratories in Aberdeen to Howie standards would be approximately £500 000 (1979 prices). Given the total number of clinical laboratories and post-mortem rooms in the UK, and the fact that the Aberdeen laboratories were not among the least easily improved, gives strong support to the argument that the costs of the Code would far exceed the benefits that might be generated. Cohen further demonstrated that there were alternative ways of achieving an equal reduction in laboratory-acquired infections which would be far more cost-effective than the Howie Code.

The main message of this study was that even a crude application of the economic approach might have led to something other than this inefficient measure being taken to reduce the particular occupational risk. That message is still true. However, since this study was undertaken other risks, in particular that of AIDS, have greatly increased among clinical laboratory workers. Thus, a re-assessment of the risks to workers would now be in order.

5.3. Discussion

Though not comprehensive in its coverage of any of the ten areas discussed, this chapter gives a flavour of how primary prevention issues can be subjected to economic appraisal. Methodological issues and attempts to overcome problems are discussed in Chapter 7. Observations are noted here on the specific question: are such studies worthwhile?

Many of the studies reviewed entailed some form of omission. Some involved only a partial analysis, e.g. the study of Loehman *et al.* (1979) which looked only at the benefit side, or they focused only on one group of benefits, e.g. Yule *et al.* (1986) who ignored all benefits of irradiating poultry bar the elimination of a single pathogen. More commonly, the studies ignored intangible costs and benefits, e.g. Schoenbaum *et al.* (1976). Indeed, the problems of considering, measuring, and valuing *all* costs and benefits may sometimes be huge. These studies demonstrate that even less than fully comprehensive studies are often useful. If, for example, analysis shows that the more easily identified, measured, and valued benefits exceed the total costs, then the efficiency of the programme is established. Inclusion of the omitted benefits can only reinforce the conclusions already drawn and is therefore not necessary. Cohen's (1983) study, which indicated that the benefits of reducing milk-borne salmonellosis could alone be greater than the cost of a ban on the sale of non-pasteurized milk, is one example of this. One key observation is that much can be learned even when such omissions are present.

Applying economic appraisal to issues where there is much epidemiological and aetiological uncertainty can highlight what additional investigation is required in order to draw conclusions about the efficiency of programmes. Goss's (1985) study, for example, produced strong evidence that reducing salt intake would be more cost-effective than screening for hypertension and administering anti-hypertensive drugs, *provided* that the claimed benefits of reducing salt intake could be shown to be valid. Evidence from trials has subsequently been accumulating to suggest the probability of significant benefits (Law *et al.* 1991). In addition to the clinical evidence that this provides, there are also immediate messages concerning the need for a change in policy away from secondary prevention (screening for hypertension and anti-hypertensive drug therapy) and towards primary prevention.

The general issue of implied values was highlighted in these studies. Muller (1980), for example, was able to quantify the price of 'freedom of choice' in the case of motorcycle helmet laws. His study may not make the decision whether or not to legislate for compulsory use of helmets any easier, but at least those who must decide can now do so on the basis of information which clearly identifies the implications of whichever course is taken. The value placed on 'freedom of choice' will be implied in whatever decision is taken. In other instances the importance of the value placed on similarly intangible costs and benefits can be identified, if not measured. Yule *et al.* (1986) showed that the ultimate factor determining the efficiency of irradiating poultry may well be the value placed on public concern over irradiation. When the evidence needed to put this study on firmer ground is forthcoming, the implied value of something as vague as public concern can be teased out.

Just why implied values are important was highlighted by Joyce, Goldman, and Grossman (1986) who argued that if society demonstrates its willingness to pay $1090 million to achieve a 10 per cent reduction in neonatal mortality by increasing the use of neonatal intensive care units, then it ought to be willing to pay at least the same amount to achieve an identical reduction via pollution control. If such a pollution control programme costs less than this amount, then those who argue that 'we can't afford it' will have to find reasons why saving a baby's life by treatment (intensive care) should be valued more highly than saving a baby's life by prevention, as this is the implication of their position.

While these studies were sometimes unable to reach firm conclusions, they could on occasion show how even the rather crude application of the principles of economic appraisal could have produced evidence which may well have changed the course of events. This was evident in the study by Cohen (1982) where it was shown that the new Howie Code of Practice was almost certainly an inefficient way of dealing with the problem of laboratory-acquired infection.

The efficiency of several preventive measures is evident from these studies. Rubella immunization, motorcycle helmet laws, fluoridation of water supplies, and banning the sale of non-pasteurized milk all produce benefits in excess of costs, while BCG vaccination of all schoolchildren and the Howie Code of Practice to prevent laboratory-acquired infection do not. In other cases the results are uncertain and normally depend on the values attached to such factors as freedom of choice or the value of time.

Economists are clearly not neutral in their desire to promote the use of economic appraisal techniques and the accompanying way of thinking. We are not unaware of our bias. However, readers may like to think about not just the problems of using economic appraisal as identified in this chapter, but the problems of not using it!

6 Case studies in secondary prevention

6.1. Introduction

This chapter reviews economic appraisals of secondary prevention. Secondary prevention is the avoidance of an impending fall in health status through early detection and treatment of incipient disease. Since secondary prevention is also commonly called screening these terms are used interchangeably.

As in the previous chapter, this selection of studies is not intended to be a comprehensive review. Selection criteria included the importance of the disease screened for, the usefulness of the results, the comprehensiveness of the methodology employed, and the significance of the issues raised. Cancer, heart disease, cerebrovascular disease, and congenital anomalies are some of the leading causes of potential years of life lost in developed countries (Romeder and McWhinnie 1977; Office of Population Censuses and Surveys 1987). While concentrating on these, we have tried to review a broad range of subjects. The ten chosen topics in screening are:

—breast cancer
—cervical cancer
—colonic cancer
—tuberculosis
—high blood cholesterol
—high blood pressure
—dental caries
—phenylketonuria
—Down's syndrome
—spina bifida

6.2.1. *Screening for breast cancer*

In the UK, North America, and Western Europe, breast cancer is a leading cause of death in women, especially between the ages of 50 and 70. Early detection and treatment might, therefore, have significant potential for extending women's life expectancy. Gravelle, Simpson, and Chamberlain (1982) addressed the question of which, if any, breast cancer screening methods would produce a net saving of health service resources, and the net health service cost per life-year gained. Their data were drawn from National Health Service clinics in London that had provided initial screening for women aged 40 and over (Chamberlain *et al.* 1975). The primary screening methods considered included not only clinical examination by a doctor, clinical examination by a nurse, mammography with the mammogram read by a junior radiologist, and mammography with the mammogram read by a senior radiologist, but also all the possible combinations of these methods, giving fifteen different possibilities in total.

As with all screening programmes, screening for breast cancer will correctly identify some people who do have disease (the true positives) and other who do not (the true negatives). Others, however, will be incorrectly identified as having disease (the false positives) or being disease-free (the false negatives). The ability of a screening test correctly to identify those who *do* have the disease is termed its *sensitivity,* and is defined as the number of true positives divided by the number of true positives and false negatives. The ability of a screening test correctly to identify those who *do not* have the disease is termed its *specificity,* and is defined as the number of true negatives divided by the number of true negatives and false positives.

Given the relatively high cost of further diagnostic tests for women with a false positive test result, Gravelle *et al.* found the specificity of the test to be crucial in determining the overall cost of screening by each method. In terms of the net health service cost per life-year gained, mammography with reading by the senior radiologist was found to be most cost-effective (£819 at 1980 prices). Other methods were found to be less cost-effective either because they were more expensive in staffing, or because they had lower specificity. None of the methods produced a net saving of health service resources.

Eddy (1985) compared other options for early detection and treatment: annual breast physical examination alone, annual breast examination plus biennial mammography, and annual breast examination plus annual mammography. The data on effectiveness were derived from the randomized controlled trial of the Health Insurance Plan of Greater New York (Shapiro *et al.* 1982) of screening women aged 50 and over. Of the methods he considered, in terms of the net medical sector cost per life-year gained, annual physical examination alone was found to be most cost-effective (US $5000 at 1985 prices).

Many of the choices to be considered in screening for breast cancer, such as the intervals between re-screening, the age or high risk groups to select, and the use of mobile screening units or hospital clinics, need further economic appraisal (Haiart *et al.* 1990). The evidence that has emerged clearly indicates that there will be no overall saving of health service resources owing to breast cancer screening. As argued in Chapter 4, however, there is no reason for necessarily expecting any saving, and assessing whether such programmes are socially efficient involves adopting a wider perspective.

6.2.2. *Screening for cervical cancer*

Cancer of the cervix uteri is a major cause of death in women and evidence has shown that screening and early treatment is effective in reducing cervical cancer mortality (Day 1989). Besides the medical costs he calculated the costs to women of attending—travelling, waiting, screening time, and biopsy time—to measure the value of the output that could have been, but would not be, produced during this time. The benefits included the value of extra output, in paid employment and housework, that would be produced by women whose cervical cancer would be prevented.

The calculations suggested that such a screening programme would produce a net saving of society's resources. The saving per women avoiding early death or disease was found to be around US $35 000 (1970 prices).

Eddy (1985) considered different lengths of interval between re-screening, in programmes for women aged 20 and over. Since epidemiological data (Guzick 1978; Eddy 1981) suggested the average time between pre-invasive and invasive cervical cancer to be around 17 years, most invasive cancers could be prevented with infrequent re-screening. Eddy calculated the net cost to the medical sector per life-year gained from screening at 5-year intervals to be around US $700 (1985 prices). This compared dramatically with the net cost of $100 000 per extra life-year gained from annual screening, over that achieved by biennial screening, owing to the substantial impact that this increased frequency would make upon costs, but not upon life expectancy. The conclusion that the marginal cost per life-year gained rises dramatically as the frequency of screening is increased has been supported by numerous recent studies including that by Koopmanschap *et al.* (1990).

6.2.3. *Screening for colonic cancer*

Even more dramatic differences in cost have been reported in a study of screening for cancer of the colon by faecal occult blood testing. Neuhauser and Lewicki (1975) considered the protocol for screening for pre-symptomatic colonic cancer that had been endorsed by the American Cancer Society. This consisted of a sequence of six guaiac tests of stools. Evidence suggested that a single test would have a 92 per cent chance of detecting cancer if it were present and the compound effect of six tests would bring a 99.9999 per cent chance. The average cost of detecting one case of cancer would be around US $2500 (1975 prices).

Their study is notable for its calculation of the extra cost of obtaining an increase in screening effectiveness. The difference in effectiveness between the compound effect of five tests and of six tests was small—99.9996 per cent and

99.9999 per cent of cancers found, respectively. Thus a population screening programme with six tests per person instead of five would increase the chances of finding cancer, if it were present, by three in a million, and the extra cost of detecting one case would be $47 million (1975 prices). Similarly, the extra cost per case detected from five tests over four was $4.7 million, from four tests over three $47 000, from three tests over two $49 000, and from two tests over one $5500. Clearly this sort of information could be brought together with information on the benefits of detecting cases and the costs and benefits of subsequent treatment, for those who have to decide whether, and how much, screening is worthwhile. It can also indicate the most effective way of spending a given budget on screening—in this case wider population coverage is likely to be more cost-effective than repeat testing in a smaller population. It also shows that even a cheap primary screening test (in this case around $2) can be very expensive in total under certain screening regimes.

Kristein (1980) estimated the net medical sector cost per true positive case detected and treated early, through single annual faecal occult blood testing among populations aged 55 and over. The cost was calculated to be at least US $3000 (1978 prices), but the social resource saving was estimated to be greater.

6.2.4. *Screening for tuberculosis*

Feldstein, Piot, and Sundaresan (1973) examined the optimal way of allocating a budget for the control of pulmonary tuberculosis (TB) in Korea. The budget was set in terms of not only the expenditure available (US $515 000 at 1964 prices), but also medical and nursing personnel, drugs, supplies, equipment, and hospital beds. They considered interventions for a range of different groups, defined by age and urban or rural residence, and the choice between screening (of those adults with chest symptoms), primary prevention (BCG vaccination), and treatment (in hospital or by domiciliary care). For most groups they found the optimal strategy to be the mass BCG vaccination of children, screening of adults with chest symptoms, and domiciliary treatment for cases found. Their study is one of the most comprehensive yet undertaken, in terms of the breadth of the possibilities considered and the carefulness with which the constraints for tackling the problem were incorporated. While their conclusions relating to Korea may not be applicable to other countries, their methodology is, and we return to it later.

Screening for TB by mass radiography had already been abandoned in the UK when Pole (1971) compared the continuation of the screening service with discontinuation and the treatment of symptomatic cases. By the late 1960s the annual incidence of TB in the UK was low (around 20 notifications per 100 000 population) and steadily declining (by around 9 per cent per year). Given this, a large, and increasing, number of people would need to be screened to find one case. The cost of treating symptomatic cases and those found by screening varied little. Pole's conclusion was that the higher net health service cost per case detected by screening did not justify the low additional benefit 'The levels of disability caused by tuberculosis are generally quite low, and the difference caused by a somewhat earlier diagnosis is probably practically negligible'. Thus he argued that the decision to abandon the service was correct, and further suggested that including the costs and benefits falling outside the health service would not diminish the case for abandoning TB screening in the UK.

6.2.5. *Screening for high blood cholesterol*

Heart disease is the leading cause of death in the UK and many other developed countries. Cretin (1977) examined the cost and effectiveness of screening 10-year-old boys for high blood cholesterol, with treatment of high levels by a cholesterol-lowering diet, to reduce, or delay, the incidence of heart disease, in the US. He compared screening with treatment of heart disease by hospital coronary care units, or mobile coronary care ambulances, in terms of cost per life-year gained. Cretin calculated the net medical sector cost per life-year gained to be US $3068 for the hospital coronary care unit, $4310 for the mobile coronary care ambulance, and between $9353 and $12 640 for screening, including the cost of the special diet (1975 prices; 5 per cent discount rate).

Berwick, Cretin, and Keeler (1981) compared different forms of screening 10-year-olds for high blood cholesterol. For males, they estimated the costs of screening and counselling per life-year gained to be US $10 660 for universal screening, $6730 for targeted screening, $5050 for school health education, and $2720 for mass media health education (1975 prices). The cost per life-year gained via mass media health education was noted to be even lower than Cretin's estimate for hospital coronary care units. They therefore concluded that mass media health education about diet may be the most cost-effective way of reducing deaths from heart disease.

In the UK, the Standing Medical Advisory Committee (Department of Health 1990) examined the cost-effectiveness of blood cholesterol testing and treatment programmes in different population groups. The cost per QALY gained ranged from £19 000 (marginal cost of drug therapy for adults receiving diet therapy) to only £44 for diet therapy alone in men aged 40–69 (1988 prices). The Committee concluded, however, that if health education could persuade every adult to adopt a recommended diet, the number offered clinical supervision because of elevated blood cholesterol concentrations would decrease by two-thirds. Screening should therefore be seen as complementary, and not an alternative, to health education.

6.2.6. *Screening for high blood pressure*

Reducing high blood pressure can prevent deaths from both heart disease and cerebrovascular disease. Stason and Weinstein (1977) compared the net health service costs and the effectiveness of different strategies in screening for hypertension (high blood pressure), including interventions for different levels of hypertension, at different ages, for males and females. Rather than measuring outcomes simply in life-years gained, they measured them in terms of quality-adjusted life-years (QALYs) gained. To adjust for quality, where adverse side-effects of treatment would be experienced, they reduced the actual number of life-years gained to reflect the lower quality of life, and where morbidity such as non-fatal cerebrovascular disease would be prevented they increased the number to reflect the higher quality of life.

The cost per QALY gained varied considerably. In the case of men with diastolic blood pressure of 110 mmHg it ranged from US $3300 at age 20 to $16 300 at age 60, and for women from $8500 at age 20 to $5000 at age 60. However, lack of adherence to anti-hypertensive medication was estimated to increase the cost per QALY gained by between 20 per cent and 100 per cent, depending on whether the medication was purchased or not.

Logan *et al.* (1981) compared two alternative strategies in screening for and treating hypertension. Their study was linked to a randomized controlled trial of screening employees in 41 business locations in Toronto. Those with diastolic blood pressure of at least 95 mmHg, or diastolic between 91–94 mmHg and systolic of at least 140 mmHg, were randomly assigned for treatment at either the workplace or a physician's office. The cost per 1 mmHg reduction in diastolic blood pressure was calculated to be Canadian $39 for the workplace option, and $67 for the physician's office option (1977 prices). The overall health system costs per person of the workplace option ($197) were around 50 per cent higher than the physician's office option ($129), but the costs to those screened and treated were nearly 50 per cent lower ($45 and $82, respectively) owing largely to the lower time and travel costs of being treated at the workplace. Probably because of the lower attendance costs, around 50 per cent more of the workplace group received drug therapy at some stage of the trial.

The findings of Logan *et al.* indicate that one way of increasing the efficiency of screening for hypertension is to reduce the costs of participating, by providing treatment at more easily accessible locations, such as the place of work. The implications for demand are discussed in Section 8.3.2.

6.2.7. *Screening for dental caries*

Geiser and Menz (1976) analysed the costs and benefits of screening school children for dental caries. They studied public dental care programmes in two cities in the US (Richmond, Indiana and Woonsocket, Rhode Island) where there was routine annual examination to detect and treat caries in its early stages.

Their objective was to estimate whether the benefits of routine examination exceeded the cost. The costs of the programme related to examination, cleaning, filling, and extraction. They could not, however, measure the value of saving teeth directly. Instead they argued that since the function of dental care is 'to enhance the appearance of the mouth and to maintain a dental structure conducive to comfort and effectiveness in chewing' and that, apart perhaps from appearance, this could alternatively be satisfied by permanent prosthetic teeth, then a minimum estimate of the value of saving teeth could be represented by the cost of replacing those natural teeth that would be lost in the absence of the programme with prosthetic teeth. Under these assumptions the benefits exceeded the costs. Thus, from society's perspective, these programmes were concluded to be efficient.

6.2.8. *Neonatal diagnosis of phenylketonuria*

Bush, Chen, and Patrick (1973) examined the net health sector cost of a programme of screening newborn infants for the inheritable disease phenyl-ketonuria (PKU) in New York State. The programme consisted of analysis of a small blood sample and, where PKU was diagnosed, treatment by a special diet. In the absence of screening, diagnosis would be delayed. If not treated in infancy PKU would cause mental handicap, possibly severe. The saving of expenditure on the institutional care of the handicapped alone was estimated to exceed the cost of the screening programme, producing a net health sector saving of $12 000 per case (1970 prices). Other benefits, such as the extra output produced at work and the humanitarian benefits resulting from the prevention of handicap would have added to the excess of benefits over costs. The programme was found, clearly, to be efficient.

This study also assessed medical consultants' ratings of the improvement in quality of life that prevention of the disability caused by PKU would bring. The average gain per case of classic PKU prevented was estimated to be 47.3 QALYs.

Thus Bush, Chen, and Patrick were able to measure the improvements in the quality of life, as well as the savings in resource expenditure, that screening for PKU could bring about.

6.2.9. *Prenatal diagnosis of Down's syndrome*

Prenatal diagnosis of congenital anomalies such as Down's syndrome does not enable the handicapped fetus to be treated. Rather it gives the parents the option of terminating the pregnancy and trying again for a non-handicapped child. While some couples who are opposed to abortion on ethical grounds would not want to consider this, there are many other couples who desire prenatal diagnosis so that they can try to ensure that none of their children is handicapped. It is these parents, and others, who are the beneficiaries of the programme.

Hagard and Carter (1976) calculated, for the West of Scotland, the costs to the health service and to the women screened of prenatal diagnosis, by amniocentesis, and subsequent terminations, of a programme to detect Down's syndrome. They then compared these with the costs that would be avoided—permanent care of the handicapped, special education, and the mother's lost work output. The avoided costs were estimated to be £10 620 per case (1974 prices; 10 per cent discount rate). The cost of detecting one case of Down's syndrome varies inversely with the risk that the woman screened will bear a child with Down's syndrome, which varies directly with her age. Hence Hagard and Carter found that there would be a net saving of society's resources if women aged 40 and over were screened, neither a net saving nor net cost if women aged 35 and over were screened, and a net resource cost if women under 35 were screened. They did not, however, include the intangible benefit of being able to terminate the pregnancy for those who had true positive results, or of reassurance to those who had true negative test results, nor the intangible costs to those who had false positive and false negative results.

Andreano and McCollum (1983) calculated the costs and cost savings to society of an amniocentesis programme for the US. Like Hagard and Carter, they found a net saving from providing the programme for all women aged 40 and over ($21 million at 1980 prices), a net saving for women aged 35 and over ($29 million), but a net cost for women aged 30 and over ($26 million). They noted that the programme would not only detect Down's syndrome, but also spina bifida, and their estimates of savings allowed for this.

6.2.10. *Prenatal diagnosis of spina bifida*

Layde, von Allmen, and Oakley (1979) examined the net resource cost to society of a programme to enable prenatal detection of spina bifida, for the US. The programme's primary screening method would be a maternal blood test, and for those found to be at high risk, a second test by amniocentesis. They estimated the lifetime, discounted, net resource cost of raising a child with spina bifida to be $68 000 (1977 prices). The cost of detecting and terminating one case of spina bifida would be around $35 000.

They also calculated the implications of the parents' subsequent decisions about their family size, having decided to terminate an affected pregnancy. Two possibilities were considered: the 'non-replacement' case in which, after the detection and abortion of the affected fetus the parents decide to have no further children, and the 'replacement' case in which the parents replace the aborted fetus by having another, presumably unaffected child. With no replacement the resource saving was the avoided cost of raising the child with spina bifida. With replacement there was, in addition, the lifetime discounted net resource contribution of the non-handicapped replacement child ($14 000), giving a resource saving per case of $82 000.

One of the present authors, Henderson (1982), estimated the costs and savings from a similar programme for the UK. With no replacement the avoided lifetime net cost of raising a child with spina bifida constituted the resource savings from the programme: around £14 000 (1979 prices). This compared with the cost of detecting and aborting one fetus affected by spina bifida of around £5700 (Department of Health and Social Security 1979). A replacement child was estimated to make a lifetime, discounted, net resource contribution of £7700 for a male. (The corresponding figure for a female was −£36 900, since output from paid employment was the only resource 'contribution' measured in this study, not, for example, output in the form of housework.)

Both these studies concluded that provision of a programme for the prenatal diagnosis of spina bifida constitutes an efficient use of health service resources.

6.3. Conclusions

The results of these studies give some direct guides to planning efficient health service resource allocation. Screening programmes for cancer of the breast, cervix, and colon are unlikely to produce overall savings of health service resources. Hence they should be thought of not as money-saving measures, but as services to be compared in terms of costs and benefits with other uses for health service resources. If screening programmes for cancer of the breast, cervix, and colon are to be undertaken, then wider coverage is likely to be more cost-effective than repeated screening of a smaller population. Initial screening for cervical cancer seems likely to produce a net saving of society's resources and, since the intangible benefits can safely be assumed to outweigh any intangible costs, such screening can unequivocally be declared socially efficient. Repeated screening at short intervals will incur a net cost, the shorter the interval, the higher the cost.

Of the alternatives for preventing deaths from heart disease by screening for high blood pressure or high blood cholesterol, none is likely to save health sector resources. Primary prevention (mass media health education about diet) and treatment (hospital coronary care units) seem more cost-effective, although better experimental evidence would be needed to draw more robust conclusions. Screening young men for severe hypertension seems about as cost-effective. Medication for hypertension may be taken up to a greater extent, and total social cost reduced, by providing more easily accessible monitoring and treatment centres, such as at the workplace.

The benefits of screening for dental caries probably exceed the costs, and routine check-ups thus seem to be efficient. The costs of screening for pulmonary tuberculosis probably exceed the benefits, at least in countries with low incidence such as the UK, and primary prevention, through vaccination, is probably a less inefficient use of health service resources.

Whether prenatal screening would save resources depends on the risk of bearing a handicapped child, but, as well as any resource saving, the intangible benefit of being able to avoid the birth of a handicapped son or daughter might be highly valued. Prenatal screening in a high risk population probably would save society's resources. Neonatal screening for phenylketonuria almost certainly saves resources as well as greatly improving the quality of life of those affected.

As important as the results is the exemplification of the methodology. In general, the broader the perspective of the question addressed, the wider the applicability of the results. Policy making should take into account the effects of screening not only on medical resources, but also on the rest of the economy, and the intangible as well as tangible costs and benefits to patients and families. It may also be helpful to know the distribution of costs and benefits by social class. The consequences of false positive and false negative test results, as well as of true positive and true negative results, should be considered. Marginal costs (and benefits) of detecting cases are more relevant than average figures, and future costs and benefits should be discounted to compare them with current resource expenditure. Finally, the results of sensitivity analysis help to indicate the importance of uncertain estimates and assumptions. The most useful studies present all this information, as Chapter 7 explains.

7 Tackling appraisal

7.1. Introduction

The previous two chapters looked at the results of economic appraisals in the areas of primary prevention and screening. Here the issues that have to be tackled to get to the results and the problems that can arise along the way are described in greater depth. The main aim of this chapter is to help the reader understand how questions of efficiency should be appraised so that the better studies can be distinguished and good practice recognized and followed.

The preliminary stage in appraisal is deciding how to set up the analysis, and one potential 'plan of action' is described in Section 7.2. First, this general scheme is elaborated. Thereafter, in Section 7.3, recurring issues, problems, and examples from studies in primary and secondary prevention are described in the context of the steps towards a complete economic appraisal.

7.2. Stages of appraisal

An economic appraisal can be broken down into a set of component parts, which is helpful for the practitioner and also serves as a useful aid to explanation. Figure 7.1 shows a plan for appraisal in diagrammatic form. This divides up appraisal into a sequence of twelve stages, which will provide the framework for the discussion.

7.2.1. Problem definition

The first stage may seem almost too obvious to warrant any discussion, but 'defining the problem' can be a very helpful exercise. This first stage asks 'What is the underlying issue or problem that has prompted the appraisal, and why is it of concern?'. Very often an appraisal is considered because a new preventive measure has been developed and a health professional wishes to know whether implementing the measure would represent a worthwhile use of resources. For example, should some newly available diagnostic test be used for the routine screening of asymptomatic individuals? Or decision makers may feel, or be persuaded, that 'more needs to be done' to avoid some particular health problem. What else could be done to prevent, say, cardiovascular disease?

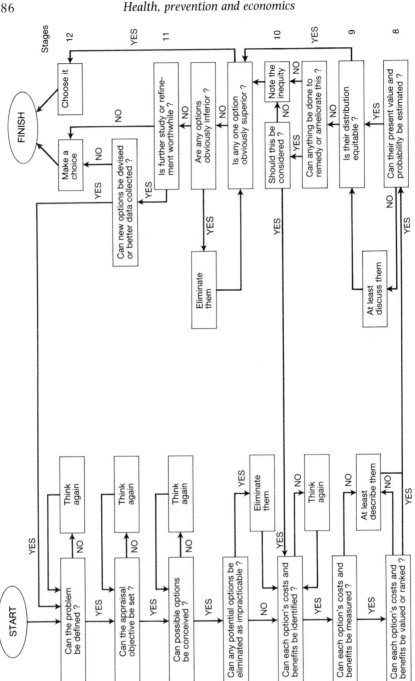

Fig. 7.1 Stages of economic appraisal. *Source:* Henderson 1985.

In general terms, the problem that most appraisals of preventive programmes seek to address is 'How can health be improved most given the particular opportunities and resources available?'. This question relates the appraisal back to two fundamental issues—maximizing health and minimizing opportunity costs. Although the particular programme under consideration may have a more limited set of objectives and constraints, it is always useful to keep relating them back to the fundamental issues. This can help to ensure that sensible options are not overlooked early on.

7.2.2. Objectives

The second stage defines the specific objectives of the appraisal, in measurable terms. For example, the objective may be to prevent the maximum number of deaths from cervical cancer given a budget of £100 million for screening. Or perhaps it might be framed in terms of producing the maximum number of life-years gained, which would give greater weight to deaths at younger ages.

Implicit in the statement of objectives is a choice between the types of appraisal described in Chapter 4: that is, cost–benefit analysis (CBA), cost-effectiveness analysis (CEA), and cost–utility analysis (CUA). CBA weighs up extra benefits against extra costs. CEA seeks the greatest effectiveness attainable within a given set of resource constraints (or the minimum cost way of attaining a specified level of effectiveness).

CUA is a variation on CEA, where the effectiveness measure is in terms of the number of quality-adjusted life-years (QALYs) gained. Bringing in quality of life has the merit of drawing attention to the ultimate objective of improving health status, and the importance of avoiding the undesirable effects of programmes, such as unnecessary treatment following false positive test results, and unpleasant side-effects of therapeutic medications, for example. Of course, it could also make the data requirements and analysis more complex.

It is also advisable to consider whose objectives are to be appraised, that is, the perspective to be adopted. Economic appraisal normally adopts the perspective of society as a whole since this makes it easier to draw conclusions concerning whether the total social benefits exceed the total social costs or *vice versa*, as explained in Chapter 4. However, the objectives of different participants—recipients, providers, and funders, for example—in the programme may differ, and it can be useful to consider whether they face conflicting incentives, which might thwart the successful implementation of findings.

7.2.3. Options

The third stage specifies the alternatives that are to be appraised. In many studies only two options are appraised: the programme *versus* no programme.

However, from a policy-making perspective it can be more useful to look at several options. This will of course depend on what opportunities are open. This in turn will be influenced by the decision-making level.

For example, the local physician who wishes to do more to reduce deaths from cardiovascular disease may face options of whether or not to begin a programme of counselling patients who smoke to help them quit; and/or screening for high blood pressure, with then a further choice amongst dietary, drug, and relaxation therapies to reduce hypertension; and/or screening for high blood cholesterol, with drug therapies and/or dietary counselling to reduce high cholesterol levels; and/or screening for high blood coagulability. There may be different ways of organizing a preventive programme. These may include options of who is to provide services: the physician, a nurse, or some other health professional. Then the programme could be based on different locations: at the physician's office, a special community clinic, or the workplace. Appraising all these alternatives will allow more careful planning of the optimum use of the physician's own time and health care resources than simply looking at one option only.

At a higher level of decision making, the government health department may be able to consider a wider range of alternatives, in addition. These could include primary prevention (such as the provision of health education programmes concerning smoking and diet, and the taxation and regulation of tobacco and particular foods) and tertiary prevention and treatment (such as coronary care ambulances and hospital coronary care units).

There are many alternatives to be considered. The wider the scope of appraisal the more confident it is possible to be that the most efficient strategy will be found. This stage gives an opportunity to try to think creatively and to come up with imaginative and perhaps novel ideas.

7.2.4. *Constraints*

The fourth stage is elimination of any options that are not feasible. Feasibility will probably be a function of several factors, but one that is common to all appraisals is a resource constraint. If a programme would use more resources than those available then it could not be implemented. Its appraisal would then be purely an academic exercise.

Another constraint may be a shortage of some necessary input to the programme—such as health professionals with specialist training. Of course such 'shortages' imply that demand exceeds supply, and this situation may be only temporary if supply can expand. Thus what is impracticable in the short term may be possible in the longer term.

Another reason for eliminating options from further consideration would be their 'inferiority'—meaning that they would be both less effective and more costly than some other option (although their inferiority may not yet be obvious at this stage).

7.2.5. *Identifying costs and benefits*

It has been mentioned that the perspective adopted is that of society as a whole. All costs and benefits should be identified and incorporated in an economic appraisal. The essence here is simple: what would have to be given up in a world with the option compared with a world without it? Similarly, what would be gained? The costs and benefits may include *direct* effects within the health care system—e.g. resources used, including the time of personnel, equipment, and consumable items—and health produced, including the reduced probability, severity, and duration of illness. The *indirect* effects are just as relevant—e.g. the resources of the recipients of programmes, their families, and society more generally, such as the time and travel costs incurred through participating in screening, and extra output produced from using healthy time gained for work. (Of course a benefit should not be double-counted by including it as both healthy time and work output produced using the same healthy time.)

The costs and benefits of programmes may be marketed—i.e. goods and services purchasable from a supplier at a market price, such as seat belts and contraceptives. The time of employees is also a marketed service, its 'price' being the wage or salary paid (plus any other employment costs). Or the costs and benefits may be unmarketed—e.g. time available for housework. Effects of programmes should not be ignored just because they are unmarketed (see Table 4.2). The dividing line between what is marketed and what is not may in any case be arbitrary. Unpaid time spent on housework produces beneficial outputs. If a home-help is hired to do the housework the benefits may be identical, but in this case a 'price' has been paid to have the service provided. But the importance and magnitude of costs and benefits are not determined by the fact that money changes hands. Appraisals should assess what resource uses are forgone (opportunity costs) or made available (benefits gained).

The costs and benefits of programmes may be tangible—e.g. using physical resources such as sphigmomanometers to measure blood pressure and drugs to control hypertension. Or they may be intangible—e.g. the anxiety provoked by a positive test result, or even just by worrying whether a result is going to be positive or negative. All good and bad effects should be enumerated in an appraisal, however intangible they may be.

7.2.6. *Measuring costs and benefits*

The next stage is to measure these costs and benefits. For many of the inputs to a programme, such as the time of health professionals, health service equipment and consumable items, it may be possible to bypass this stage and go straight on to valuing them in monetary terms—using their market price. Other inputs, such as recipients' time, may be unpriced and may need to be measured (e.g. hours spent) before being valued (at an appropriate hourly rate).

The most difficult problems are normally in measuring the outcomes. The units of measurement will vary from programme to programme—e.g. numbers of unwanted pregnancies avoided, smokers who have quit, years of life gained, and so forth. At this stage the problems of determining such numbers—i.e. of measuring effectiveness—are not problems peculiar to economic appraisal, but would be encountered in any evaluation of a programme's outcome. Epidemiologists are professionals at designing studies to assess outcomes objectively, and interpreting outcome data (Barker and Rose 1979). Uncertain estimates of outcomes may later (Section 7.2.8) be subjected to sensitivity analysis to assess whether their reliability is crucial or unimportant.

If no objective measures are available, outcomes may still be measured quantitatively, using ratings given by experts based on their professional judgements. Such methods may be criticized as being 'unscientific', but in the absence of better measures they may be useful, particularly if professionals who are closely involved in the programme are thereby made to consider more carefully how the effectiveness of a programme should be evaluated.

In CUA the outcomes are measured in QALYs gained. QALYs have been estimated in research studies that have asked health professionals and members of the general public to make assessments of the value of changes in health. The assessments sought may be direct—e.g. asking people to rate health status on some sort of scale (like a thermometer)—or indirect, via people's preferences for trading-off health changes against other things.

The trade-offs used may realistically reflect the choices that some individuals occasionally have to make in health care—e.g. whether to accept a treatment that will either kill or cure them or not to accept it and remain in a state of impaired health, or whether or not to accept a treatment that will definitely cure them but which will also reduce their life expectancy. The size of the risk, or the reduction in life expectancy, that people would be prepared to accept to gain an improvement in health in such circumstances, gives an indication of the subjective value they attach to the health improvement. These two types of trade-off have been built up into techniques for assessing QALYs, and are known as the 'standard gamble' and 'time trade-off', respectively. Some results of their use are reported in Section 7.3.5.

7.2.7. Valuing costs and benefits

If the resources used, or made available, by a programme have prices in competitive markets, where there are no significant externalities or other distortions, then it may be inferred that their price reflects their value (see Chapter 3). Prices taken from uncompetitive markets may have to be adjusted, the adjustment being downwards to take out any element of 'overpayment' because of monopoly profit, or upwards in the case of 'underpayment' where there is monopsony (monopsony being the demand-side equivalent of monopoly).

The values of unmarketed resources have to be calculated by other means. It is here that economists have been criticized for 'knowing the price of everything and the value of nothing'. The charge is rather unfair, though, since the figures that should be incorporated in an economic appraisal are individuals' own values of the consequences of programmes, as revealed in either the choices that they make or their directly expressed preferences.

Choices can reveal the values of marketed goods and this can be observed in the way that people choose different levels of consumption in response to price changes. This can allow the change in consumer's surplus to be calculated as a measure of the cost or benefit of a price change (see Section 5.2.7).

Often in the appraisal of preventive programmes, there are no relevant data to make such calculations because the inputs and outcomes whose values are being sought are not marketed. In such cases the appraisal may have to make use of special data collection exercises. These may range from simple questionnaires, to a few programme participants, to full-scale national sample surveys. For example, the latter has been undertaken on behalf of the UK Department of Transport to estimate the value that road users would place on reductions in the risk of death and injury in motor vehicle accidents. Some of the results are reported in Section 7.3.6.

7.2.8. *Discounting and sensitivity analysis*

The notion of time preference was explained in Chapter 4—i.e. that people prefer benefits sooner and costs later—and, therefore, to reflect their *present value*, future costs and benefits are discounted. The choice of discount rate remains a subject of controversy among economists. Essentially, the controversy surrounds the issue of whether to adopt the rate that prevails in financial markets, or, since most economists agree that this rate is 'contaminated' by factors such as taxes, externalities, and transient macro-economic objectives of the government of the day, by how much to depart from this rate.

A simplistic solution to this problem is to go for consistency rather than theoretical exactness. One American author has suggested that every appraisal should use a 5 per cent discount rate (Russell 1986) which would make comparing appraisals easier. In fact, in the 1980s the UK Treasury advised that a 5 per cent discount rate should be used. In April 1989, however, they revised this to 6 per cent for monetary values, but recommended a lower rate for utility measures such as QALYs (HM Treasury 1991).

Use of a range of different rates would help to show whether the results were materially affected by the choice of rate. Chapter 4 has explained about the use of such 'sensitivity analysis'.

If the true value of some figure to be used in an appraisal is not known with precision, but is believed to lie within some specified range, the analysis can deliberately use several values—e.g. 2 per cent, 5 per cent, and 10 per cent discount rates—to see what difference they make. If the overall conclusions are unaltered then the lack of precision is unimportant. If the conclusions are changed—i.e. are sensitive to the choice of value used—then greater precision would be desirable, and thought might be given to refining the analysis, or collecting better data, to increase the reliability of the estimates. Although greater precision may be desirable, it may be impracticable, or disproportionately costly to achieve. If so, then at least the sensitivity analysis makes clearer the circumstances under which the conclusions would be changed and by how much they would be affected.

If there is a good data base from which to draw estimates then it may be possible to calculate statistical confidence intervals. These are often expressed as ranges within which there is 95 per cent, or 99 per cent, confidence that the true value lies. Such calculations obviously give a better indication of the size of the uncertainties involved in the analysis. However, they do rely upon the existence of a good data base, which may not always be available. Hence there is likely to be a place for both calculation of confidence intervals and sensitivity analysis.

7.2.9. *Equity*

It has been mentioned that the perspective adopted in CBA is that of society as a whole and that conclusions are based on whether the total social benefits exceed the total social costs or *vice versa*. The reason for using this criterion is that if the benefits are greater than the costs then, logically, it would in principle be possible to compensate those who bear the costs, by redistributing the benefits, so that no one need bear any costs. Clearly, this would be an ideal arrangement. In practice it may be difficult to arrange such redistribution.

More importantly, there are value judgements to be considered in deciding who ought to benefit, and by how much, and who ought to bear costs, and how much. This is where principles of equity may be brought in. Particular groups in society may be felt to merit special consideration. Benefits accruing to, or costs falling on, these groups may be deemed to be more important than to other groups, for reasons of fairness, justice, desert, or need.

For example, accessibility to screening clinics may be given special significance in poor areas, because access costs may be considered to be a greater burden on poor people than on rich people. Therefore special arrangements may be considered for poor areas, such as bringing screening services nearer by, say, using mobile vans or setting up special community clinics. Or again, higher taxes on particular products that would form a much greater proportion of the weekly income of a poor family than of a rich family may have the effect of widening inequalities in disposable income: this has been one of the main arguments put forward against steep increases in taxes on tobacco, for example.

Assessment of the distributive consequences of programmes may find them to be equitable or inequitable, as well as efficient or inefficient. Programmes may ultimately be judged against both these criteria. If they are inequitable this may either count as a point against their implementation, or lead to them being redesigned to ameliorate their inequitable effects.

7.2.10. *Superiority and inferiority*

If all the consequences of each option are valued in monetary terms then it will be possible to sum all the values to produce a net total for each option. If the net total is negative then the costs exceed the benefits and the option is inefficient. If the net total is positive then the benefits exceed the costs and the option is efficient. If a choice has to be made between the options (e.g. if only one may be implemented) then the superior option is that with the largest positive net total.

Assessing the most efficient option is more difficult in CEA and CUA, where the costs and benefits are not measured in commensurable terms. If one option is found to be superior to all the others—meaning that it has both greater effectiveness and lower costs—then that is clearly the one to choose. Inferior options—having both lower effectiveness and higher costs—are to be rejected. Choosing beyond that is dealt with under Section 7.2.12.

7.2.11. *Refinement*

One reason for refining an appraisal has already been referred to—that sensitivity analysis may have indicated that greater precision of estimates would be desirable. Another may be that a new option can be envisaged that might, for example, combine elements of options already appraised, so homing in on an option that might have still greater benefits or lower costs. Yet another may be that events have moved on since the appraisal was begun and new possibilities, constraints, or influences have emerged. If relevant data can be found then refinement of the original appraisal could be worthwhile.

7.2.12. *Choice*

If one option emerges as superior then that is the one to choose, on efficiency grounds. Of course it is possible that it may be so inequitable that this overrides its efficiency, and that some more equitable but less efficient option is preferable. The efficiency sacrificed in such a case would be the 'price' of greater equity.

It is often tempting to try to make the choice among the options on the basis of ratios of benefit, or effectiveness, or QALYs gained, to cost. However, there are pitfalls to this approach. In theory it is possible to manipulate any ratio by changing the numerator and denominator by the same amount: a ratio of £300/−£150 is greater than a ratio of £250/−£100, for example, yet the only difference between them is that the numerator of the second is £50 less and denominator £50 more. Although these two ratios may differ, the *profit* is the same: £150 in both cases. Calling a consequence of an option a 'negative benefit' instead of a 'cost' can have just this effect of changing the ratio of benefit to cost, without changing its overall value (see Section 4.4.2). Thus it is not possible to choose on the basis of ratios of benefit, or effectiveness, or QALYs, to cost if there are inconsistencies in the way in which particular consequences have been dealt with across different options. But if consistency has been maintained across all the options then they may be ranked in terms of such ratios.

A second problem is that it is then tempting to choose the option at the top of the ranking. However, there is nothing in the theory of economic appraisal to say that only the top option should be chosen. It could be equally valid to choose several options, in rank order, or even all the options. In essence, the problem is that CEA and CUA do not give any indication of how much should be spent in total—they only show which options are more, and which less, efficient. In CBA any option(s) for which the numerator exceeds the denominator should be chosen.

A third problem is that selecting options in rank order may leave some of the available budget unused. If so, then it is possible that a selection of options other than in rank order that did more nearly exhaust the available budget could provide greater total benefits. This is unlikely to be a problem in practice provided that the option that is 'missed off the end', using this selection method, can be scaled down so that it uses up the remaining budget.

Of course a decision is needed at some stage in CEA and CUA to determine how big the budget should be. This means that a value judgement is required as to whether the effects are worth, or not worth, the costs of achieving them. The advantage of CBA is that it explicitly addresses that very issue.

7.3. Issues

In this section important issues that come up in economic appraisals are illustrated with examples from studies whose results were reported in Chapters 5 and 6, as well as others not previously discussed. The framework used for the discussion is the plan described in Section 7.2.

7.3.1. *Problem definition*

Sometimes the problems that policy recommendations seek to address do not relate back to the fundamental issues of maximizing health *and* minimizing opportunity costs. For example the Howie Code (see Section 5.2.9) sought only to reduce risks of infection in laboratories—it did not consider opportunity costs. When the costs of implementing the recommended risk reduction methods were later estimated, doubt was cast on the wisdom of the code under prevailing circumstances. Overall benefits can only be maximized if costs are considered as well.

7.3.2. *Objectives*

The objectives of individuals can differ from those of society. This is likely when the actions of individuals have significant external effects for others, as in the case of immunization against communicable disease. From an individual's perspective the benefits (reduced risk to themselves of acquiring the disease) may not be sufficient to outweigh the costs (time, trouble, dislike of injections, and risk of side-effects). On this basis they may decide against inoculation.

From a societal perspective there are additional benefits, through the reduction in risk that one individual's immunization confers on others by reducing the spread of disease. From a collective perspective the total benefits may outweigh the total costs, implying that greater levels of inoculation would be desirable than individuals may decide upon. Even subsidizing the cost, so that it is free to those who receive it, may not be sufficient incentive to produce optimal uptake rates.

Fine and Clarkson (1986) applied this theory to pertussis (whooping cough) immunization where very serious side-effects are possible (although rare) with the vaccine currently available. They showed that under plausible values for the efficacy of the vaccine and perceived risks, individuals will choose a socially sub-optimal level of uptake. Their calculations could enable the threshold to be determined below which the risks, or at least perceived risks, would have to be reduced to bring uptake up to the optimal level.

Weighing up benefits and costs is the objective of CBA. But the effect of external benefits and costs can be that the optimal outcome differs with the perspective adopted. Successful implementation of the socially efficient outcome may depend upon knowing the cost–benefit balance from other perspectives.

7.3.3. *Options*

Policy makers may assume that specific regulation of hazardous or preventive products is the only option for their control. However, other options are supply-side intervention in the market, e.g. taxes and subsidies, or demand-side intervention to make consumers better informed, e.g. health education.

For example, in the US there was pressure to do more to reduce deaths among youths from motor vehicle accidents related to alcohol consumption. Legislators considered the option of raising the legal drinking age to reduce deaths. This would affect all youths, even those who did not drive. Saffer and Grossman (1986b) showed that the same effect could be achieved by raising the taxes on beer (see Section 5.2.8). This would affect all ages, however, not just youths, although reduced consumption may have beneficial effects at other ages, too. Thus a tax increase was established as another effective option.

Gravelle, Simpson, and Chamberlain (1982) appraised fifteen different screening methods for early detection of breast cancer. These consisted of all the possible combinations of physical examination by a doctor and/or nurse, and mammograms read by a junior and/or senior radiologist (see Section 6.2.1). Even a small set of options can be increased by considering combinations and permutations.

Very often it may be possible to consider options of primary, secondary, and tertiary prevention, and treatment. Feldstein, Piot, and Sundaresan (1973) appraised options not only of screening for tuberculosis, but also of primary prevention by BCG immunization, and of treatment of symptomatic cases (see Section 6.2.4).

7.3.4. *Constraints*

In CEA there is often a fixed resource constraint, within which effectiveness is to be maximized. Stason and Weinstein (1977), in their study of screening for hypertension (see Section 6.2.6), specified an objective of gaining the greatest possible increase in QALYs from spending $1 million on hypertension. They calculated the proportion of a $1 million budget that should be devoted to initial screening, repeat screening, treatment, and efforts to reduce drop-out rates and increase adherence to medication.

Sometimes monetary cost will not be the only constraint that will limit the size of a programme. Feldstein, Piot, and Sundaresan (1973) set the objective in their study of the Korean tuberculosis control programme (see Section 6.2.4) as being to maximize the reduction of death, disability, and lost output, subject to the constraints of US $515 000 (1964 prices) for total expenditure, $130 000 for supplies and equipment, 83 million minutes of doctor-time, 130 million minutes of nurse-time, 22 million minutes of technician-time, and 830 000 hospital bed-days. They calculated how the benefits could be maximized by pursuing different options to varying extents, subject to these six constraints.

7.3.5. *Measuring costs and benefits*

Intangible costs such as pain, suffering, and anxiety are clearly difficult to measure. Sometimes, however, it can be sufficient to weight these costs, rather than to try to value them, for the purposes of choosing between a set of options. Mooney (1982), for example, considered the cost-effectiveness of different ways of screening for pre-symptomatic breast cancer, using data from a health service clinic in Edinburgh, Scotland. Six possible screening regimes were considered, consisting of combinations of mammography, thermography, and one or two clinical examinations. As well as measuring the resource costs, the anxiety costs attributable to the different screening methods and diagnostic biopsy rates for the regimes were assessed, and a relative anxiety weight given to each regime. Of the options considered, mammography plus one clinical examination was concluded to be the most cost-effective. Thus in this case it was possible to include the cost of anxiety without putting an explicit monetary value on it.

In their study of tuberculosis control in Korea (see Section 6.2.4), Feldstein, Piot, and Sundaresan measured the benefits in four alternative ways: avoided life-years of temporary disability (bed confinement); avoided life-years of permanent impairment through reduced lung function; avoided premature deaths; and avoided losses of marketed output. Rather than use only one of these measures, or try to combine all four into a single weighted measure, they calculated the optimal strategy for maximizing each benefit measure independently. They argued that it was for responsible government officials or public health administrators ultimately to judge which strategy would maximize social welfare.

In fact they found that the differences in strategy implied by switching from maximizing one measure to maximizing another were relatively small. Hence the most efficient way of allocating a given quantity of resources to the reduction of a particular disease could be determined without putting monetary values on the benefits, or even relative weights on different benefits, in this case.

In a British study, Parkin and Moss (1986) estimated the marginal benefits of different screening regimes for cervical cancer in England and Wales. There is debate about the frequency with which screening should be undertaken in the UK and there have been calls for intervals to be reduced from 5 years to 3. Parkin and Moss showed that resource inputs of '1000 units' (costing approximately £10 000 at 1986 prices) would produce benefits of 21.8 life-years gained under 5-yearly screening, but only 15.5 life-years gained under 3-year screening. Their results also varied with assumptions about the natural history of the disease and screening attendance rates, but under all sets of assumptions the benefits achieved by the same resources were lower for the more frequent screening. This is a good example of the common finding that as programmes are expanded marginal benefits diminish.

Bush, Chen, and Patrick (1973) measured the improved quality of life at different ages that would be produced by neonatal screening and treatment for phenylketonuria (PKU) (see Section 6.2.8). They asked medical specialists to predict the levels of disability that would ensue, with and without treatment, and to rate the desirability of different levels of disability on a scale from 0 (equivalent to death) to 1 (equivalent to full health). One year with a disability level rated at 0.25 can be termed 0.25 QALYs, equivalent to 3 months with full health. They estimated that the prevention of one case of classic PKU would produce a gain of 47.3 QALYs (see Fig. 7.2).

Sackett and Torrance (1978) measured the preferences for different levels of quality of life of a stratified random sample of the general public of Hamilton, Ontario, using the time trade-off method. They asked people what fraction of a year of full health would be worth giving up to avoid some particular disability

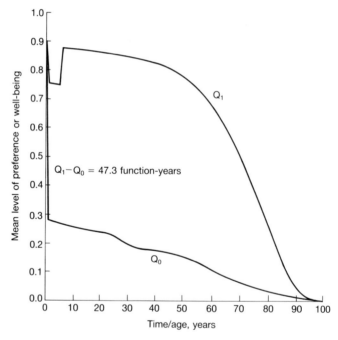

Fig. 7.2 Quality of life. Mean level of well-being over time for classic PKU with and without treatment using consultants' value set. Upper line, representing treated cases, depicts initial dysfunction imposed by diet during first 6 years, then gradual decrease in mean function imposed by general mortality rate. Lower line (untreated cases) shows lower levels of function and also higher mortality rates experienced by severely retarded. *Source*: Bush, Chen, and Patrick 1973.

for a year. They found that women equated one year with a mastectomy for treatment of breast cancer to 0.48 years with full health (i.e. 0.48 QALYs). If a screening programme could prevent the need for mastectomy it would bring a gain of 0.52 QALYs per woman, in their view. This figure could then, in principle, be used to make comparisons with the outcomes of other ways of using available resources, so that the maximum benefits could be aimed for.

7.3.6. *Valuing costs and benefits*

The value of resources such as time available for unmarketed activities have to be estimated using proxy methods. For example, Schweitzer proxied the value of time spent on housework by the prevailing market wage rate for women (see Section 6.2.2). Among the resource costs and resource benefits of screening for cervical cancer, he included the value of extra future housework by women in whom cervical cancer would be prevented. In addition the costs to the woman of participating in screening were calculated—it was estimated that travelling, waiting, and the procedure itself would take around 1.5 hours, while a diagnostic biopsy following a positive screening test would involve 2 hours of the woman's time. This was costed at the average hourly female wage rate, whether or not the woman was in paid employment, as a measure of the opportunity cost of her time.

Sometimes it is possible to estimate a minimum value of the benefit of a programme. If this is found to exceed the cost then the programme is efficient (and a more accurate estimate of the benefit may not matter). Geiser and Menz (1976), in their study of the costs and benefits of screening for dental caries (see Section 6.2.7), adopted this approach. They argued that, with the possible exception of appearance, prosthetic teeth fulfilled all the functions of natural teeth. Therefore a minimum estimate of the benefit of screening for dental caries could be represented by the cost of replacing those teeth that would be lost through caries, in the absence of screening, with prosthetic teeth. Since this measure of the benefit exceeded the cost of screening they concluded that the programme was efficient.

Consumer's surplus lost or gained is theoretically the most accurate measure of cost or benefit (see Section 5.2.7)—i.e. the amount that consumers would have been willing to pay over and above the amount that they actually had to pay. It can only be observed, however, when demand curves are apparent. Ippolito and Ippolito (1984) estimated, for the US, consumers' reduced willingness to pay for cigarettes after official warnings about the health risks were issued in 1964. Their analysis, after controlling for other influences, suggested that the immediate impact of the warnings was that demand for cigarettes shifted back and consumption fell by 17 per cent. The ratio of previous willingness to pay to the post-information willingness to pay gave an estimate of consumers' valuation of the health risks. The authors used this information to calculate consumers' valuation of a life-year gained to be around $10 000 (1980 prices).

Since tobacco is an addictive good, however, could consumers adjust their consumption by the amount they really wanted to? In the short term they may reduce only a little (while wishing they had never started), but in the long run they may quit. Hence true consumer's surplus may be difficult to measure in the case of addictive goods.

Sometimes the benefits of programmes that save lives are measured as the future earnings of those whose lives would be extended. This may be an estimate of their opportunities to consume marketed goods and services, but it under-estimates the total value of the reduced mortality risks.

For example, Forester *et al.* (1984) (see Section 5.2.8) estimated the benefits of reductions in road accident deaths in the US. They presented several estimates: one showed tangible benefits to other members of society only—the future output of those whose deaths would be postponed, less their future consumption; a second showed tangible benefits to society as a whole—the future output without deducting consumption; and a third showed estimates of willingness to pay—these exceeded the estimates based on future output, as might be expected.

Cohen *et al.* (1983) (see Section 5.2.4) analysed various benefits of preventing salmonellosis, one of which would be a reduced risk of death. As a minimum they incorporated the 'value of life' used by the UK Department of Transport (DTp) in appraising road safety projects—£100 000, based largely on forgone earnings. By contrast, Jones-Lee *et al.* (1985) conducted a study of people's willingness to pay to reduce risks of death and injury from road accidents. In their national sample survey people were asked how much extra they would be prepared to pay to travel by safer means of transport. The answers indicated that people were prepared to pay much more than would be inferred from the DTp figures. In fact they indicated a 'value of life' of around £1.5 million (1983 prices). In general, estimates that base benefits only on avoided losses of future output will be too low.

7.3.7. *Discounting*

Jackson (1987), in an article on fluoridation to prevent tooth decay (see Section 5.2.5), claimed that if fluoridation cost £0.20 per person per year then it would cost £14 over a 70-year lifespan. This ignores discounting. The present value of the cost of fluoridation is lower, since resources that do not have to be used now can be invested meantime. Discounting £0.20 at a 5 per cent rate over a 70-year lifespan gives a present value of only £4. Thus the over-estimate from ignoring discounting can be very significant in the case of long-term horizons.

7.3.8. *Sensitivity analysis*

Often measures of costs and benefits have to rely upon estimates or assumptions that may be unreliable. A prudent response to this problem is to try out alternative estimates and assumptions.

An example of this sensitivity analysis is given in Figure 7.3. It shows the benefits of a prenatal screening programme for open spina bifida, under different assumptions about: the likelihood of the 'replacement' of a terminated pregnancy; the level of 'psychological' (intangible) costs; and the discount rate (Henderson 1982) (see Section 6.2.10). Also shown is the cost of providing a

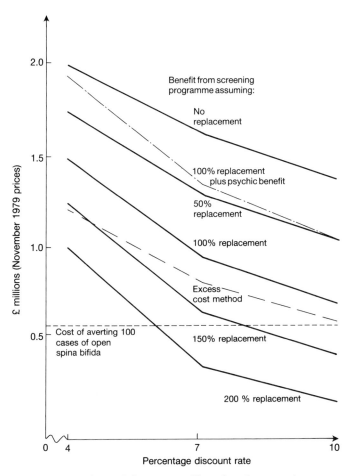

Fig. 7.3 Sensitivity analysis of the costs and benefits of a screening programme for open spina bifida. *Source*: Henderson 1982.

screening programme. Sensitivity analysis can indicate where uncertainty is relatively most important to the conclusions, thereby suggesting priorities for further research, or it can indicate that despite the uncertainty the conclusions are relatively robust. In Figure 7.3 it can be seen that the benefits exceed the costs under all but extreme assumptions.

Another good example is given in the study of the cost-effectiveness of different methods of promoting smoking cessation by Altman *et al.* (1987) (see Section 5.2.6). They showed the costs per quitter of three options under all the plausible assumptions about the effectiveness (quit rates) of the methods. Results are depicted in Figure 7.4. This sensitivity analysis indicated that only under extreme assumptions did the self-help kit fail to be the most cost-effective option. The conclusion was therefore insensitive to errors in the measured estimates of effectiveness, and confidence in the conclusions was increased.

7.3.9. *Equity*

It is often assumed that increasing the taxation of tobacco is a regressive policy, i.e. hits the poor harder than the rich. This is assumed because it is observed

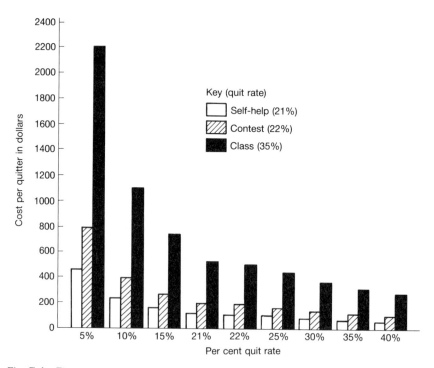

Fig. 7.4   First year costs per quitter under different quit rate assumptions (excluding developmental costs). *Source*: Altman *et al.* 1987.

that smoking rates are higher among the poor than the rich. However, this ignores the fact that the response to price changes may differ between different income groups—the poor may respond more and suffer less from a price rise than the rich. Little is known about how responsive different income groups are to price changes. Townsend (1987) has provided some estimates for the UK. She estimated that unskilled manual workers would spend less on tobacco as a result of a price rise, while higher social classes would spend more in total. Hence tobacco price rises may not be so regressive as many suppose.

Rich, Glass, and Selkon (1976) undertook a cost-effectiveness study of screening schoolgirls, in an English city, for asymptomatic bacteruria. Dipslide urine testing by the girls themselves, or a parent, at home yielded 70 per cent coverage, at a cost per girl screened of £0.26 (1973 prices). Testing at school achieved 85 per cent coverage, at a cost per girl screened of £0.55, or with extensive efforts to reduce non-attendance 96 per cent coverage, at a cost per girl screened of £0.77. For the first 70 per cent of the group the home dipslide was clearly the most cost-effective method. The extra cost of increasing coverage beyond the 70 per cent achieved by the home method was £1.93 per extra girl up to 85 per cent coverage, and from there £2.45 per extra girl up to 96 per cent coverage (Glass 1979).

It was found, however, that while coverage for the home dipslide method was 70 per cent averaged over all the girls, of girls whose fathers were unemployed or in unskilled manual jobs only 58 per cent were screened, whereas 84 per cent of girls whose fathers were in non-manual jobs were screened. If health service decision makers had an objective of equity across social classes they may be prepared to pay higher costs per girl to achieve higher rates of coverage in which there was a more equitable social class composition. Such equity is clearly not costless.

7.4. Conclusion

This chapter has tried to indicate what constitutes good practice in economic appraisal. The plan of action described in Section 7.2 shows the steps that a full appraisal should go through. As explained above there are many issues that pose problems, both methodologically and empirically. However, the case studies show that most problems are capable of resolution, following the example of the better studies.

8   Demand and consumption

8.1. Introduction

Section 3.2.1 explained that a demand curve normally slopes downward from left to right, reflecting the fact that when price is high a smaller quantity of the good is demanded than when price is low. Economists are also concerned with how responsive demand is to price changes and use the concept of *elasticity* to measure this. The demand for a good is said to be 'price elastic' if proportionately small changes in price cause proportionately large changes in demand and 'price inelastic' if the opposite is true. For example, if a 20 per cent rise in price causes a 10 per cent fall in the quantity demanded (price elasticity of -0.5), then demand is said to be inelastic. If a 10 per cent rise in price causes a 20 per cent fall in the quantity demanded (price elasticity of -2.0), then demand is said to be elastic. In these examples the negative signs indicate that price and demand move in opposite directions.

Demand is not, of course, influenced solely by price. There are other measures of elasticity to reflect responsiveness of demand to these other influences. Income elasticity measures the responsiveness of the quantity demanded to changes in income, and advertising elasticity to changes in the amount of advertising. Cross-price elasticity reflects how responsive the quantity demanded of one good is to the change in price of another, for example how the demand for tea responds to a change in the price of coffee. Many demand studies present their results in terms of these elasticities.

Elasticity values are succinct ways of summarizing information on the extent to which the quantity demanded will change in response to various potential influences. Some of these will be under the control of policy makers. For example, the government can raise or lower price by means of taxes and subsidies. It can reduce or prohibit advertising and affect people's disposable income through income taxes and allowances. The elasticity values indicate the effect of such potential changes on demand.

The methodology for demand analysis is well developed and many goods that have preventive or hazardous qualities have been subject to them. In this chapter we review four areas under two broad headings:

(1) market goods:
  (a) the demand for cigarettes;
  (b) the demand for alcohol;

104

(2) preventive medicine:
   (a) the demand for breast cancer screening;
   (b) the demand for hypertension screening and treatment.

The studies discussed here all represent the application of conventional demand analysis to preventive or hazardous goods. The fact that the market goods in question have attributes which affect health was largely incidental to the analyses. This means that although the results are of interest to the study of prevention the methodology is not unique to it. Chapter 9 takes a deeper look at some characteristics that distinguish preventive/hazardous goods from ordinary commodities, i.e. goods that do not affect health. It argues that these differences often justify a different approach.

8.2. The demand for preventive/hazardous market goods

In this section we look at the demand for market goods which happen to have the attribute of increasing the risk of future illness and death, as well as other risks (such as fire in the case of cigarettes and accidents and violence in the case of alcohol). The studies to be discussed examine the extent to which factors such as price, income, and advertising influence demand, in much the same way as do studies of goods which do not affect health. One difference is that some investigate the effect of health education, but as will be shown in Chapter 9, health education can be viewed as another form of advertising.

8.2.1. *The demand for cigarettes*

The demand for cigarettes is a well researched area for a number of reasons. First, there is the belief that reductions in cigarette consumption will lead to dramatic reductions in morbidity and mortality (Doll 1983). This in turn will have a major impact on such things as costs to health services and sickness absence from work (see Section 3.3.3). Another reason concerns the huge revenue generated from tobacco taxation. Dramatic changes in the demand for cigarettes can have major consequences for government finance.

Empirical investigations of the demand for cigarettes go back a long way (Stone 1945). Since the link between smoking and ill-health was established in the mid-1960s there have been many more studies, particularly to examine the preventive potential of fiscal policies. Investigations have focused on four principal issues:

(1) the effect of changes in price on aggregate demand;
(2) the effect of advertising by tobacco companies on aggregate demand;

(3) the effect of anti-smoking publicity and other forms of health education on aggregate demand;

(4) the effect of changes in income on aggregate demand.

Elasticity is measured as the proportionate change in aggregate demand resulting from a proportionate change in the variable of interest (price, income, or whatever). Elasticities have been measured for three of the above variables, but not for anti-smoking publicity because it has been difficult to establish any relationship between the amount of publicity and cigarette consumption. Investigating responsiveness to marginal changes in publicity will have to wait until the existence of any causality can be more firmly established.

8.2.1.1. *Price*   The results of studies of the price elasticity of demand have varied according to the methodology used and to the way other variables that affect demand were dealt with. There does not appear to be any consistent variation according to when or where the studies were undertaken.

Estimates of the price elasticity of demand from nine studies are given in Table 8.1.

If price elasticity is near zero, as was found by Atkinson and Skegg (1973) in the case of men, then demand is largely unaffected by changes in price. The further is the estimated price elasticity from zero, the more responsive is demand to changes in price. Price elasticity of −1, for example, means that a 10 per cent rise in price would cause a 10 per cent fall in demand. This is significant from the point of view of government revenue. Price elasticity is smaller than −1 in all estimates, which implies that governments considering raising tobacco duty can be confident that reductions in revenue from some

Table 8.1   Price elasticity of demand for cigarettes

Study	Elasticity
Stone (1945)*	−.50
Sumner (1971)*	−.24
Hamilton (1972)#	−.51
Russell (1973)*	−.60
Atkinson and Skegg (1973)*	−.34 for women, 0 for men
Peto (1974)*	−.07
Fujii (1980)#	−.45
Witt and Pass (1981)*	−.32
Lewitt, Coate, and Grossman (1981)#	−.25 for teenagers

Note: * = United Kingdom, # = United States

people smoking less, or quitting, will be more than offset by the higher tax per packet paid by those who continue to smoke.

8.2.1.2. *Advertising* There is considerable controversy surrounding the relationship between advertising and the demand for any good. Both Schmalensee (1972) and Lambin (1975) have concluded from extensive research over a range of goods that advertising has little if any effect on aggregate demand. This conclusion has been taken up by the UK Tobacco Advisory Council (1981) who argue that cigarette advertising affects choice of brand only (i.e. market share), but has no influence on the amount smoked. The view that advertising does not affect aggregate demand is also expressed by the Advertising Association (Waterson 1981), but, interestingly, only in the case of cigarettes and alcohol.

Most demand studies support this view. (See, for example, Fujii 1980; Hamilton 1972; Johnson 1980; or Metra Consulting Group Ltd 1979.) One notable exception is the study by McGuinness and Cowling (1975) which found a significant advertising elasticity of 1.4 in the short term and 2.8 in the longer term, the positive sign indicating that advertising and aggregate demand move in the same direction. The explanation for the often indiscernible effect of advertising may be the integral health warning that is a mandatory feature in many countries.

Despite weak evidence of any association between advertising and aggregate demand, most countries have banned cigarette advertising on radio and television. In the UK, the Royal College of Physicians has called for a complete advertising ban except at point of sale (Royal College of Physicians 1983).

8.2.1.3. *Health education* As with advertising, it is notoriously difficult to isolate the effects of health education and anti-smoking publicity from other influences. Warner (1977) found that the cumulative effect of persistent publicity was substantial and estimated that without such publicity per capita consumption in the US would have been some 20 per cent to 30 per cent higher than it was in 1975. Most studies, however, have tended to focus on consumer reaction to shock effects such as the US Surgeon General's Report (1964), which first officially recognized the link between cigarette smoking and ill-health, or that of its UK counterpart, the Royal College of Physicians' Report (1962).

Estimates vary but seem to indicate that, in the US, the fall in demand resulting from the report was in the order of 5 per cent (Warner 1977, Fujii 1980; Hamilton 1972; Lewitt, Coate, and Grossman 1981), and that the effect of the publicity rapidly wore off. Roughly the same 5 per cent fall in initial demand with rapid return to pre-report levels was found in several UK studies (Sumner 1971; Atkinson and Skegg 1973; Russell 1973; Peto 1974). In

Switzerland, however, Leu (1984) found that the effect of major publicity events was permanent, reducing consumption by some 11 per cent.

8.2.1.4. *Income*   Income elasticity is of interest in so far as, if positive, the effect of rising incomes could offset the effects of rising taxation or greater anti-smoking publicity. Unlike tax or publicity, though, income is not a specific policy tool which can be used to influence demand. Income does not appear to have a dramatic effect on the demand for cigarettes. Estimates vary from about 0.3 (Witt and Pass 1981) to 0.6 (HM Treasury 1980).

8.2.2. *The demand for alcohol*

Like tobacco, alcohol is responsible for much preventable morbidity while at the same time being an important source of government revenue. Accordingly, there is no paucity of studies on the demand for alcohol, although unlike smoking which is felt to be bad *per se*, alcohol only poses health problems when abused.

Demand studies in this area have tended to focus on price. The effect of advertising on aggregate demand has also been investigated, but to a much lesser extent. The effects of health education appear to have been omitted from economic demand models (Godfrey 1986) perhaps because non-economic studies (e.g. Plant *et al.* 1979) suggest that health education campaigns do not appear to have a significant influence on consumption.

8.2.2.1. *Price*   The demand for beer, wine, and spirits is normally analysed separately because the consumption of each varies among different groups in the population. Demand studies in this area also trace back to Stone (1945). Estimates of price elasticity of demand from six studies are given in Table 8.2.

These results are consistent in finding the demand for beer to be price inelastic, but there is no such consistency in the case of wine or spirits. Lau's (1975) study is based on a different population from the others, but it is interesting to note that the Treasury estimates, in the case of wine and spirits, are out of step with the other three UK studies. If the Treasury estimates are correct, and elasticity is really greater than unity, then the government will lose revenue if tax on wine or spirits is increased. If the other estimates are correct then there would be a revenue gain from a tax increase.

8.2.2.2. *Advertising*   Since the general effects of advertising on the demand for all goods is not well established, it is not surprising that evidence of the effect of alcohol advertising on aggregate demand for alcohol is patchy and controversial. As a general conclusion from those studies that have attempted to explore this area (e.g. Hamilton 1972; Bourgeois and Barnes 1979) it would appear that there is no significant relationship between the two.

Table 8.2 Price elasticity of demand for alcohol

Study	Elasticity		
	Beer	Wine	Spirits
Stone (1945)*	−.73		−.72
Comanor and Wilson (1974)#†	−.56	−.68	−.25
Lau (1975)‡	−.03	−1.65	−1.45
McGuinness (1980)*	−.30	−.17	−.38
H.M. Treasury (1980)*	−.20	−1.30	−1.10
Walsh (1982)*	−.13	−.38	−.45

Note: * = United Kingdom, # = United States, ‡ = Canada, † = Short run

8.2.2.3. *Income* All of the studies whose findings were reported in Table 8.2 also estimated income elasticities. These are shown in Table 8.3.

It appears that beer is income inelastic, but wine and spirits may well be income elastic. This implies that a 10 per cent rise in income causes a rise in demand for beer of less than 10 per cent, but a rise in demand for wine and spirits of more than 10 per cent.

Table 8.3 Income elasticity of demand for alcohol

Study	Elasticity		
	Beer	Wine	Spirits
Stone (1945)*	.14		.54
Comanor and Wilson (1974)#†	−.18	.41	.18
Lau (1975)‡	.20	1.43	.68
McGuinness (1980)*	.13	1.11	1.54
H.M. Treasury (1980)*	.70	2.50	1.80
Walsh (1982)*	.13	.50	1.20

Note: * = United Kingdom, # = United States, ‡ = Canada, † = Short run

8.3. The demand for preventive medicine

The previous sections looked at the demand for market goods which have attributes capable of affecting health. Conventional demand analysis of the effect of changes in price on demand could be readily applied because the goods have prices attached. In this section we consider the demand for medical services which are often either provided at zero price to the consumer or for which some form of cost-sharing arrangements exist.

8.3.1. *The demand for breast cancer screening*

There are dangers in applying conventional demand analysis to priced or unpriced medical services because it is often not possible to separate the *demand* for these services from the decisions of the suppliers. The demand for screening services, however, is more likely to be based on consumer sovereignty because, first, those who come forward for screening do not do so in response to being unwell and, second, the decision to be screened is more likely to be patient-initiated than are decisions to consume most other medical services.

As was explained in Sections 1.4 and 4.4.1, consumers incur numerous non-monetary costs even when a good or service is zero-priced. Following economic theory, the lower these costs the greater should be the expressed demand for screening. Thus, if screening were available at a local clinic rather than at a more distant location, individuals would incur lower costs in terms of travel fares, lost earnings, lost time from other activities, and inconvenience. The lower the costs the greater the expected level of expressed demand for the service. It would also be predicted that if the costs incurred increased with the distance travelled then demand would decline as distance increased.

A study of attendances at a NHS breast cancer screening clinic in England supported this theory. Gravelle and Simpson (1979) found an inverse relationship between the attendance rate and both the home to clinic distance and the time and travel costs of those attending the clinic.

Also in the UK, one of the present authors and colleagues examined the demand for a mobile breast cancer screening service (Haiart *et al.* 1990). They expected demand to vary inversely with access costs. Using distance as a proxy for access costs, they indeed found that a 10 per cent increase in distance brought about a 2.4 per cent reduction in attendance rates.

Haiart *et al.* (1990) also predicted that demand would vary positively with income and wealth. It was not, however, possible to measure income directly. Employment was used as a proxy. The study found that a 10 per cent increase in female employment rates in the relevant age band was associated with a 4.1 per cent increase in attendance rates.

The implications for policy from studies of the demand for screening are clear. Conventional demand theory is borne out, signifying that reducing costs to consumers will increase the uptake of screening services. Such reductions can involve either subsidizing consumers for travel and time costs or bringing services closer to consumers. If the cost of providing mobile vans is less than that of providing fixed-site clinics, and if such a service is shown to be no less effective in detecting pre-symptomatic cancers, then the Haiart *et al.* study will have shown mobile vans to be the more cost-effective form of screening and an important means of providing incentives for greater uptake.

Haiart *et al.* also examined the effect of 'advertising'. In addition to posters around the town, information leaflets were delivered through letter boxes in selected districts. This adversising, however, produced no discernible effect on uptake, after controlling for distance and socio-economic class.

8.3.2. *The demand for hypertension screening and treatment*

Logan *et al.* (1981) compared two alternative strategies in screening for and treating hypertension in Toronto, Canada. One group was provided with treatment at the workplace while the other had to go to a physician's office for treatment. Thus the latter group incurred higher costs for any given quantity of service. As might be expected they consumed less medication than the workplace group.

In terms of the supply and demand curves of Section 3.2.1, the two groups could be thought of as facing two different supply curves while having the same demand curve. This idea is expressed in Figure 8.1, which shows a single demand curve for reduction of hypertension, but two supply curves—one where treatment is available at less cost at the workplace, and the other where treatment is available at greater cost at the physician's office. Note that the vertical axis measures cost per *unit of output* (reduction in blood pressure) *not* cost per unit of activity (screening, medication, etc.).

Logal *et al.* found that the mean reduction in diastolic blood pressure after a year was 12.1 mmHg for the workplace group and 6.5 mmHg for the physician's office group. The cost per mmHg reduction at the workplace was C$39, represented by $W in Figure 8.1, and C$67 for the physician's office group, represented by $P.

Similar results were found by Keeler *et al.* (1985) who looked at the effect of different types of insurance on reductions in blood pressure. Here, people with high blood pressure faced different costs according to whether their insurance covered the full cost or was one with a cost-sharing arrangement. As expected, the amount of treatment consumed varied according to the proportion of the cost that had to be borne by the patient. There was a corresponding variation in outcome. The reduction in diastolic blood pressure in the full coverage group was significantly greater than in the partial coverage group at the end of the experiment ($p < 0.05$).

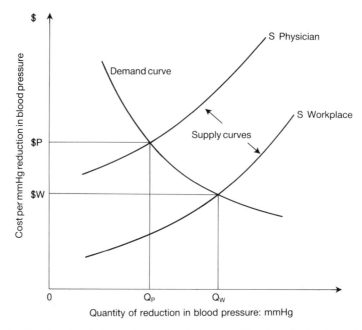

Fig. 8.1   Supply of and demand for secondary prevention in reducing hypertension.

    These studies on treatment for hypertension show the importance of the
distribution of costs between the consumer and others (provider, insurance
company, or the state) on expressed demand. In the study by Logan *et al.*
overall costs to the health service were greater at the workplace, but because
the costs per person to those receiving treatment there were so much lower,
the resulting higher level of demand led to greater reductions in hypertension,
making the workplace option the more cost-effective of the two. The Keeler *et
al.* study does not allow the same conclusion to be drawn since the costs per
unit reduction in hypertension are not given. The study does, however, show
the extent to which 'charges' act as a deterrent to use and to effectiveness.

8.4. Discussion

The studies discussed in this chapter have viewed the demand for goods that
affect the risk of future illness or injury as responding to essentially the same
influences as other goods. The demand for screening and hypertension
treatment were shown to be as influenced by *price* (access costs) as that for
cigarettes or beer, although all are relatively 'price inelastic'. The demand for
both cigarettes and alcohol was found to be unresponsive to advertising.

Interestingly, Haiart *et al.* also found the uptake of breast cancer screening to be unresponsive to advertising. With regard to income, cigarettes, beer, and screening are shown to be income inelastic, while the demand for wine and spirits appears to be more responsive to income.

Such information is of obvious values for planning and policy making. The low price elasticities for cigarettes and beer suggest that increasing taxation on these goods will be a good source of government revenue but will have a more limited effect on reducing levels of consumption. This could, however, have important equity implications since consumption of both cigarettes and beer is higher among lower socio-economic groups. On the other hand, lowering access and other costs for breast cancer screening or hypertension treatment can be an effective way of increasing uptake rates. The evidence on advertising elasticities is less conclusive, but it suggests that advertising has little effect on total demand. This implies that advertising bans may be less effective in reducing consumption than proponents of such bans might hope, and less effective than manipulating price.

The assumption that the factors which influence the demand for these goods are the same as those which influence the demand for goods that do not affect health is open to question. Chapter 3 explained that demand is determined by the amount of utility which a good is expected to yield in consumption. But can the utility that a consumer expects to gain from being screened for cancer be looked upon as being similar to that expected from buying a pair of shoes? After all, no one derives pleasure in the usual sense of the word from attending a screening clinic. If demand is determined by utility, and the utility from prevention is different, might not the demand for prevention require a different type of analysis? The following chapter explores this possibility.

9 Preventive behaviour: a closer look

9.1. Introduction

Price, income, and advertising are all factors which are expected to alter the demand for any good be it preventive, hazardous, or neutral in terms of its effect on health. Thus there is no reason why the demand for screening cannot be analysed in the same framework as the demand for shoes, as was seen in the previous chapter. Estimates of the price, income, and advertising elasticities of demand for screening are valuable pieces of information.

As was the case in Chapter 8, the focus of this chapter is on the demand for prevention, but here it is based on a view which takes as its starting point the fact that there is something fundamentally different in the reasons for demanding screening as opposed to shoes. The nature of the utility yielded by goods affecting health will be shown to be different from that of goods that do not affect health, suggesting that the demand for prevention will require a separate type of analysis if consumer behaviour in this area is to be better understood.

This chapter reviews some of the major contributions by economists on this issue, showing particularly how theories on the demand for prevention developed from theories on the demand for health care. From this base a new approach will be presented. Consumer behaviour with regard to the demand for goods affecting health will be shown to be identical to what is called 'preventive behaviour' or, more generally, 'health behaviour' in socio-psychological analyses. Similarities between the economic approach and the socio-psychological will be highlighted.

9.2. The market for prevention

When examining the demand for prevention it is apparent that such demand is for a host of different goods and services, some of which will be provided in the formal health care sector (vaccines), others in private markets (fluoride toothpaste), and others in markets with some form of government control (alcohol). Some will be tangible goods (fire alarms), others intangible (exercise). Some will be consumed solely for their effects on health (vitamin tablets), while for others the effect on health will not necessarily be the major consideration in the decision to consume (wholemeal bread). Furthermore, prevention implies not only greater consumption of those things which are 'good for you', but, equally, avoidance of those things which are 'bad for you'. The problem in defining the market appears almost insurmountable. There is, fortunately, one factor common to all of the above. In every case consumption of the product or service *alters the individual's risks of future ill-health.*

Here actual alteration of the risk of future ill-health is used to define the market for prevention, rather than individuals' perceptions of whether particular behaviour and consumption is preventive or otherwise. By this view, someone who demands a good which they believe to reduce the risk of ill-health but which does not, is not demanding prevention. Equally, someone who demands a good that does reduce risk is demanding prevention even if they are unaware of the effect of the good on risk.

The importance of this distinction will become evident later in this chapter. Initially the argument concentrates on the fact that most preventive and hazardous goods are perceived as being preventive or hazardous. While some forms of prevention may be consumed for non-health reasons, most are at least partly consumed because individuals want a higher level of health. We can say that the demand for prevention is largely derived from the demand for health; and while everyone wants to be more healthy not everyone is equally willing (or able) to pay for improved health. Some of the reasons for differing demand for health will be investigated later in this chapter, as will the reasons why some seemingly obvious prevention is not perceived as such by the consumer. First, a brief history of the development of this type of approach is useful in understanding the main messages which follow.

9.2.1. *A development of the demand for health approach*

The idea of viewing the demand for prevention as being derived from the demand for health grew from the seminal work of Grossman (1972) who examined the factors affecting the demand for health care (i.e. treatment and cure). Previous studies in this area had focused on such factors as the cost of health care and distance to the facilities. Grossman, however, argued that analysis of the particular variables that affect the demand for health care would be better and more accurately studied within a much broader analysis of the nature of health itself. With the recognition and acceptance of the Grossman approach, subsequent investigators argued that, since the only significant difference between the consumption of health care and the consumption of prevention is in the timing of the consequential change in health state, the Grossman approach should apply equally well to the demand for prevention. It will be argued below that while such an analogy is valid and provides many valuable insights into our understanding of preventive behaviour, much of the published literature has perhaps drawn too close a parallel with health care and consequently many important aspects have been omitted in several of the attempts to explain and predict preventive behaviour.

9.2.2. *The Grossman view of the world*

Grossman's theory of the demand for health care drew heavily on the earlier work of Becker (1964). Conventional economic theory views production as being the activity of firms and consumption that of households. Becker radically departed from this by arguing that households or individuals should not only be seen as consumers, but also as producers who produce 'fundamental commodities' using market goods and their own time as inputs in a production process. For example, instead of regarding individuals solely as consumers of food—a consumption good—individuals could also be seen as producers who use food as one of the factor inputs of a production process which combines various other inputs (such as wine, candles, etc.) with their own time to produce the commodity 'dinner'. The value of this approach is that food is no longer regarded as being demanded for its own sake. Rather, it is now a producer good whose demand is derived from the demand for 'dinners' in much the same way as the demand for looms is derived from the demand for cloth. If through theory and empirical investigation the factors which determine the demand for the fundamental commodity can be identified, then the demand for the factor input will also be largely explained.

Following this approach, Grossman postulated that health is a fundamental commodity which is produced by individuals using health care and their own time as the principal inputs. Health care fits very well into this framework, since unlike almost all other goods, it does not directly yield utility—except perhaps to those few unfortunates with Munchausen syndrome!

In Grossman's model, individuals are viewed as having a stock of health that depreciates, over time, at a rate which increases beyond some certain age. Death results when the stock falls below some critical level. In any time period, however, new 'investments' can be made—in other words more of the stock can be produced—by combining health care and own time.

When analysing why people demand health, Grossman postulated that there are two distinct (and in his model totally independent) reasons why people want to be healthy. First, any increase in the amount of 'healthy time' will allow for increased productivity at work, giving an increase in earnings. Second, all consumption during 'healthy time' gives more utility than when the individual is unwell. Just think how much more you enjoy your holiday in Greece if you avoid 'holiday tummy'.

Grossman's model predicts how the demand for health care varies with age, education, wealth, and income. Despite the radical nature of the approach the results produced few surprises, essentially showing that individuals are capable of making efficient choices without any form of outside interference. This is based, however, on an assumption that individuals are fully aware of their existing level of health stock, the rate at which it depreciates, how to produce more health, and can perceive their optimal level of health.

The model has been criticized for being a complex analysis which offers little in the way of implications for health policy (see, for example, Cullis and West 1979). However, if individuals can be shown to be efficient producers of health when they have the relevant information on the nature of health-producing inputs and how they can be combined, then a clear policy implication emerges. For if it is believed that such knowledge is not present, then a shift of public policy to the provision of health information rather than the provision of more health services might be justified.

One major advantage of the Grossman approach is that it places the relationship between health care and health in a more realistic perspective, suggesting that the importance of other factors may overshadow the effects of health care on the health of the individual. Later in this chapter we will see the extent to which the same thing can be said about the effects of prevention on health.

Despite any weaknesses, Grossman's model is something of a landmark. His introduction of the concept of health as a durable capital good has shifted the focus of economic research away from examinations of individual variables related to the demand for health care into a much broader analysis of the nature of health itself. It is this shifted focus that permits investigation into the demand for prevention, derived also, at least partly, from the demand for health.

9.3. The demand for prevention after Grossman

Grossman's pioneering work has been extended by many since its introduction in 1972 (see Grossman 1982). Here we concentrate on those with implications for prevention, drawing on three important works.

9.3.1. *Cropper*

In the conclusion to his 1972 paper, Grossman acknowledged that his model contained a number of simplifying assumptions and pleaded for further developments in the area—in particular, for the role of uncertainty to be introduced. Cropper (1977) took up the challenge and presented a 'Grossman-type' model whose main feature was a departure from the assumption of perfect knowledge on the part of individuals. The model has the added advantage of providing a better framework for separate analysis of specifically preventive inputs into the health production process.

In Cropper's model, the stream of utility from consuming during 'healthy time' is temporarily interrupted by illness and permanently interrupted by death. While consumption clearly will not cease during illness the assumption is that the utility it yields is effectively the same as if no consumption took place. Investment in the stock of health is therefore undertaken in order to increase the expected utility from consumption.

Unlike the Grossman model, illness is analysed as a random event whose probability depends on the level of the health stock. When illness occurs, curative investments will be made in order to resume the utility stream. Preventive investments, however, are made in order to increase the level of health stock and hence reduce the probability of future illness. This probability cannot be reduced to zero. Cropper thus neatly separates preventive health care, which is non-random, from curative health care, which is a random event. The focus of her investigations is on the preventive component.

Initially, Cropper's model assumes that the time of death is independent of the level of health stock and is known with certainty. While no less unrealistic than the Grossman assumptions, it leads to radically different predictions. In Grossman's analysis, investments in health are made mainly in response to illness, and illness is positively correlated with age. Thus the demand for new investments will increase with age. In Cropper's model, and owing to the random nature of illness, the non-random preventive investments in health will tend to decrease with age since investments made later in life yield returns over a shorter period than those made earlier. This issue of the timing of illness, as compared with the timing of prevention, is an important point as will be seen shortly. When Cropper's assumption of death's being independent of the stock of health is dropped the results are unfortunately less clear.

Aside from its importance in separating prevention from curative investments, Cropper's approach is also valuable in that by treating illness as a random event, preventive health care becomes dependent on *expected future utility*. Individuals can place very different values on future utility even if the value they place on current utility is the same. This concept of delay affecting the value of utility will shortly be argued to be a more important determinant of the demand for prevention than Cropper allows.

Finally, Cropper's work is important in that she considers *dis-investments* in health stock due to choosing a risky occupation. In her model, individuals trade-off higher wages against an increased probability of dying. Interestingly, Cropper's model shows that once exposed to the dangers, individuals who remain in risky occupations are behaving entirely rationally. The importance of introducing hazards in addition to preventive inputs is an important expansion of the analysis.

9.3.2. *Ippolito*

The concept of hazardous consumption has been extended by Ippolito (1981) who examined consumption patterns of goods that increase the risk of dying, and particularly those situations in which the hazardous nature of a good only becomes known after consumption has begun. In Ippolito's analysis, the cost of a hazardous good includes not only its purchase price, but also has an element reflecting the cost in terms of reduced length of life. While traditional economic theory predicts changes in demand due to changes in price, Ippolito showed how these changes are also dependent on the nature of the hazard in question. The reaction to constant hazards (i.e. those that have a fixed probability of death per unit consumed), will differ from that when the risk is cumulative. Similarly, the reaction will differ in the case of a risk of immediate death, compared with delayed death, even if the probability of death is the same in both cases.

Ippolito's contribution is valuable in that it moves away from the very generalized models of demand toward analysis of individuals' behaviour relative to single consumption issues. The focus on the nature of particular hazards will be argued, below, to be of paramount importance in explaining the demand for particular goods. The main weakness of Ippolito's approach concerns its focus solely on death. Indeed, goods that alter the risk of illness without affecting the risk of death are excluded from the analysis. A further weakness concerns Ippolito's neglect of the subjective valuation of future utility alluded to above.

9.3.3. *Muurinen*

The two developments of the basic Grossman model have mainly concerned the dropping the assumption of perfect knowledge and certainty. Muurinen (1982) argued that although such developments were important, there remained some fundamental weaknesses in the underlying Grossman framework which required improvement.

Foremost among these weaknesses was Grossman's treatment of the two reasons for demanding health—more healthy time leading to more work (wages), and increased utility of consumption—as separate and rival hypotheses. Muurinen argued that this separation was artificial as the demand for both types of benefit from increased health is simultaneous.

Perhaps of greater importance, though, was Muurinen's introduction of the concept of use-related depreciation. Now the stock of health not only depreciates with time as the individual ages, but also depreciates according to how intensively the individual 'draws' on it. Thus unhealthy living explicitly reduces the stock of health more quickly than does healthy living.

Furthermore, Muurinen's analysis introduces other non-health stocks that individuals also possess (i.e. wealth and education) and postulates that the rate at which individuals draw on their stock of health depends on the relative size of that stock as compared with the others. This helps to explain why the health affecting behaviour of the poor and uneducated often differs from that of the wealthy and well-educated.

Interestingly none of Muurinen's alterations leads to radically different predictions from those of the original model. Her results, however, appear to be drawn from a more realistic base and do not depend on the restrictive assumptions of the Grossman model.

9.4. Where has this taken us?

The models described are all valuable contributions to an understanding of the demand for prevention. There are, however, three remaining problems in all of them.

9.4.1. *The general nature of ill-health*

One problem common to all of the above models is their reliance on the well/ unwell (or in the case of Ippolito, alive/dead) dichotomy. While there are certain advantages to maintaining such a level of generality, the approach forfeits the insights that could be gained by analysing the *nature* of particular outcomes. Ippolito comes closest to overcoming this by introducing the notion of the nature of a hazard (e.g. constant versus cumulative risk) but the nature of her only *outcome*, death, is the same in all cases. None of the models account for outcomes of differing severity. Since many preventive measures are taken against specific outcomes, it is likely that the perceived severity of that outcome will be a factor affecting demand. The duration of that outcome is also important, but this aspect can be handled by any of the above models.

9.4.2. *The timing of the benefits of prevention*

In all of the above models the utility from the consumption of prevention is that which comes from consuming other goods and services while healthy, and from the wages from production made possible by being healthy. The problem with this view is that the benefits of prevention *only* arise in the future, long after the preventive consumption takes place. It cannot account for utility which consumers may derive between the time that the preventive measure is taken and the time when the unwanted outcome would otherwise have occurred. In other words, in none of these models can prevention give 'peace of mind' or the perception of security. These would seem to be important aspects to try to incorporate in any model of prevention.

9.4.3. *Prevention for other reasons*

All of the above models focus on a demand for prevention as prevention. In other words prevention is undertaken specifically because the consumers want to increase their stock of health. Goods that may be only incidentally preventive, i.e. which are mainly consumed for non-preventive reasons, do not fit well into the models. In fact, people who demand (say) wholemeal bread because they simply prefer its taste over that of white bread, but who are unaware of the link between dietary fibre and risk of bowel disorders, would not be trying to increase their stock of health when they demand wholemeal bread. The demand for this product could not, in this example, be described as being derived from the demand for health. Such non-preventive reasons for undertaking prevention can be of importance in explaining, predicting, and attempting to modify preventive behaviours.

The following section departs from the household production approach to introduce some new elements to the analysis. Before proceeding, however, it should be noted that many disciplines other than economics have analysed prevention. Indeed, the psychological perspective predates the economic, and considerably more investigations have been undertaken from that standpoint.

9.5. A non-economic view: a psychological model of the demand for prevention

In much the same way that economic demand models for prevention developed around a seminal work on the demand for health, many psychological prevention models (see, for example, Becker and Maiman 1975) developed from the more general 'Health Belief Model' which was first formulated by Rosenstock (1966). Instead of the 'demand for prevention' referred to above, the Health Belief Model speaks of 'health behaviour' and 'health affecting behaviour'. This different jargon arises from the different perspective, but the similarities are clear.

The Health Belief Model has three essential elements which together explain health behaviour. (For comparative purposes we will refer to this as preventive behaviour.) The first concerns the individual's subjective state of 'readiness to take action'. This depends on perceptions of both the likelihood of a particular illness or injury occurring, and perceptions of the severity of that outcome, should it arise. The second element concerns the individual's own assessment of the potential benefits of adopting a particular preventive behaviour, weighed against the 'barriers' involved (such as cost, effort, or pain). Finally, a stimulus is required to set off the behaviour. The stimulus can be either internal, like a bodily feeling, or external, such as a health education campaign.

This view of preventive behaviour might appear to have little in common with the economic demand models described above. In fact, when stripped of jargon, the two approaches can be seen to have much in common, though there is one fundamental difference between them. The psychological models focus on specific behaviours undertaken to prevent specific outcomes, while the economic models focus on a more general desire to prevent ill-health.

The model which follows incorporates elements of both the economic and psychological models, though it is essentially an economic approach. Its main focus is on the *anxiety* associated with any threat. This model provides an alternative theory of preventive behaviour to the other models, but is not intended as a contradiction of them.

9.6. A new model of preventive behaviour

9.6.1. *Principles*

Uncertainty was introduced into the Grossman–Muurinen framework by making illness and death random events dependent on, but not wholly determined by, the level of health stock. The lower the stock of health, the greater the probability that the individual will suffer some unspecified illness or die. Clearly, many preventive measures are undertaken in order to reduce overall levels of risk. As was shown above, much can be gleaned by analysis at such a level of generality. However, it is also apparent that illness is not a homogeneous event. Many preventive measures are undertaken to reduce the risk of specific unwanted outcomes, leaving other risks unchanged. In fact some forms of prevention may be so strongly related to a specific outcome that they become hard to describe in a generalized human capital framework at all.

In conventional demand theory, a consumer will consume a particular unit of a good if the marginal utility yielded by that unit is of greater value than the cost of acquiring it. If the focus of analysis shifts from a general view of avoiding illness and death to the nature of specific unwanted outcomes, then the willingness to bear the marginal cost of a preventive action will depend on the perceived dis-utility of *that* outcome (i.e. the perceived utility from avoiding it). Sackett and Torrance (1978) have demonstrated that the dis-utility of different illness conditions can vary markedly, even over illnesses of equal severity and duration. If the values attached to two outcomes differ, then the demand for preventive measures to avoid them will also differ, even when the marginal costs are the same. This suggests that analyses which view the dis-utility of illness solely in terms of the loss of production and consumption benefits, may not be sufficient to explain the demand for all forms of prevention. A reassessment of the nature of the utility derived from prevention is in order, but before doing so, it is worthwhile clearly stating the assumptions and definitions underlying all that follows.

1. All preventive actions precede the outcomes that they are intended to

prevent. There is thus always a lag between the time when the preventive action is undertaken, and the time when the outcome is avoided.

2. Few unwanted outcomes are certain to arise in the absence of prevention, and few are certain to be avoided with prevention. There is some probability between 0 and 1 of any outcome arising.

3. Prevention can play one (or more) of three roles. First, it can reduce the probability of an outcome occurring, second, reduce the severity of that outcome and third, reduce the duration of the outcome.

4. The concept of 'risk' can be defined to include all of the three dimensions above. Though the term 'risk' is often used as a synonym for 'probability' we prefer to use it in its wider connotation. In the analysis which follows, risk refers to probability, severity, and duration combined (or to use the jargon, the expected value of the loss).

5. If prevention is defined in terms of reducing levels of risk, then many 'preventive' actions may not be undertaken for preventive reasons at all.

9.6.2. *Prevention goods and hazard goods*

At the beginning of this chapter, the difficulties of specifying the goods and services to include in a 'market for prevention' were highlighted. The common factor in all the examples listed was that in every case consumption alters the individual's risk of future ill-health. Therefore:

—A *prevention good* is any good or service, the consumption of which reduces the risk of ill-health.
—A *hazard good* is any good or service, the consumption of which increases the risk of ill-health. (Cohen and Mooney 1984.)

The vague prevention market, spoken of earlier, can now be formally defined as the market for prevention goods and hazard goods. Since hazard goods are the obverse of prevention goods (or are negative prevention goods) we will use the term 'prevention goods' to refer to both, unless a specific hazard good is being discussed.

The first thing to note when viewing the demand for prevention in these terms is that the reasons for consuming prevention goods may have nothing to do with the definition. By the definitions above, someone who consumes a good which they believe is reducing the risk of ill-health, but which is not, is not consuming a prevention good. The individual's demand for this good is not considered as a demand for prevention. Equally, someone who consumes a good that does reduce risk is consuming a prevention good even if the consumer is unaware of the effect of the good on risk. In this case the individual's demand for the good *is* part of the demand for prevention.

9.6.3. *The utility from prevention*

In the household production models described earlier, illness breaks the stream of healthy time and stops or reduces the flow of utility. Since prevention seeks to avoid this, the utility from prevention is defined as the utility that would otherwise be lost. This view of utility from prevention is too restrictive and is insufficient fully to explain much, if not most, preventive behaviour.

There are two types of utility overlooked in the view adopted above because of two fundamental shortcomings:

1. In all the household production models utility arises at the time when the unwanted outcome is avoided. Unsuccessful prevention therefore yields no utility at all in these models. In an article on the value of life, Schelling (1968) raised the point that if individuals are aware that they face a high risk of dying then:

... the pain associated with the awareness of risk—with the prospect of death—is probably often commensurate with the cost of death itself. . . . This anxiety is separate from the impact of death itself. It applies equally to those who do not die as to those who do, to people who exaggerate the risk of death as much as if the estimates were true. It counts, and is part of the consumer interest in reducing the risk. (pp. 145–146)

It follows that any preventive measures taken to reduce the risk of dying, even if the perceived risk is exaggerated or imagined, will yield utility from the reduced *anxiety* that accompanies the risk. There is no reason to suppose that this will be true only in the case of the risk of dying, but will also apply in cases of risk of all unwanted outcomes. Such utility is not accounted for in the above models.

2. A second shortcoming of the models reviewed is their concentration on the preventive nature of prevention. It must be remembered that much prevention is undertaken for reasons unconnected with prevention. Since high-fibre cereal is associated with lower risk of bowel disorders, then high-fibre cereal is a prevention good. The demand for high-fibre cereal is part of the demand for prevention. Nevertheless, to many people high-fibre cereal is a tasty and enjoyable product which may be demanded partly or even wholly for its hunger- and taste-satisfying attributes. The utility from prevention goods derived from their non-preventive attributes is not accounted for in the above models.

It appears, then, that prevention goods have two distinct types of attributes (i) that of reducing risk and (ii) that associated with the use value of the good. Each yields a distinct type of utility. Lancaster (1966) has developed a theory in which utility is seen as being derived from the attributes of goods, rather than from goods themselves. Following this we can say that all prevention goods by definition contain attributes that affect risk. If it is assumed that anxiety is a function of risk (Mooney 1977), then these risk-affecting attributes can also be viewed as attributes affecting anxiety. Since lower anxiety is preferred to higher anxiety, there is a utility gain associated with the consumption of prevention goods (and a utility loss associated with the consumption of hazard goods).

There are two points to note from this special type of utility which, borrowing from Weisbrod (1964), we call *utility-in-anticipation*. First, it is yielded immediately after the prevention takes place and continues as a stream of utility until the time when the outcome was anticipated. Second, it is dependent on the anxiety associated with the *perceived* risk, and with the *perceived* effectiveness of prevention in reducing that risk. As in Schelling's case, the actual level of risk and the true effectiveness of that preventive action, are not relevant in themselves.

In the human capital approach, though, utility arises only at the time that the outcome is avoided. Since one rarely knows what would have otherwise happened after a preventive action is taken, this notion of avoided loss of utility is insufficient on its own to explain all preventive behaviour. The benefits of prevention do not all arise at the time when the outcome is avoided. A fire extinguisher does not only yield utility when a fire actually occurs, but also yields utility-in-anticipation from the knowledge that it will be available in case of fire.

The second type of attribute may not be contained in all prevention goods, but is certainly contained in most—and always in the case of hazard goods. Clearly prevention goods such as vaccines yield no utility in the usual sense of the term since no one derives any pleasure from vaccination. The only type of utility yielded in the case of such perfect prevention goods is utility-in-anticipation. But for many prevention goods there is a use value. The utility derived from *this* attribute is here called *utility-in-use*.

Total (or net) utility is the sum of the two. Both forms of utility can be positive, zero, or negative. Economic theory predicts that consumption will take place if the (net) utility provided by any unit of a good exceeds its cost.

Utility-in-use is an important concept in attempts to alter the demand for prevention. It is, however, a conventional economic concept and will not be explored in detail here. Utility-in-anticipation, on the other hand, is a less well-established concept and requires further explanation.

9.6.4. *The determinants of utility-in-anticipation*

Utility-in-anticipation can be defined as the difference between the dis-utility of the initial anxiety associated with the original level of risk, and the dis-utility of the final anxiety associated with the post-prevention level of risk.

As stated earlier, few preventive measures are 100 per cent effective so the final risk level and the associated anxiety are rarely zero.

Clearly the difference between the two levels of anxiety depends on how effective the prevention good is in reducing risk. However, since demand is subjective, the amount of utility-in-anticipation that a good yields depends on the *perceived* effectiveness not on the actual effectiveness of the good. Someone who is unaware of a particular good's preventive effectiveness will derive no utility-in-anticipation from consuming it. Someone who believes that a particular good reduces risk, even when it does not, still receives utility-in-anticipation from its consumption.

We must then ask what it is that determines the initial level of anxiety. Two elements combine to determine this. First, there is the value of the loss associated with the unwanted outcome, and, second, there is the degree to which the individual suffers dis-utility because of risk.

9.6.5. *An explanation of terms*

The analysis which follows will make use of three terms which need to be defined.

9.6.5.1. *Expected loss*   Expected loss is identical to risk, as defined earlier. It is the product of the perceived severity and duration of an outcome, and the perceived probability that the outcome will occur. Note that in both cases, and as with perceived effectiveness of the prevention good, expected loss is subjective.

9.6.5.2. *Present value of expected loss*   One thing that is certain about the expected loss is that it is not 'expected' until some time in the future. Rational people will prefer to postpone losses for as long as possible. In other words, the present value of the expected loss (which is of course a negative value) is lower the farther in the future it is expected. As indicated in Section 4.4.5, economic analysis uses discounting to express all future losses (or gains) in terms of their present values. Such values depend on: first, the length of the period between the present and when the loss is expected to occur; second, the rate of discount used.

9.6.5.3. *Risk aversion*   An identical present value of an expected loss can generate different anxiety levels according to how averse individuals are to risk. Some individuals dislike taking risks more than others. (In economic terms they would be willing to pay a higher price to avoid the same risk than would others, other things being equal.) For others still, some risks can even give a positive thrill.

The link between greater risk aversion and a higher yield of utility-in-anticipation is best explained by means of an example. Take the case of a 'pure' prevention good (i.e. one that has no use value and thus only yields utility-in-anticipation) and further assume that the good is perceived to be 100 per cent effective (i.e. after consumption, risk, and the associated anxiety, are reduced to zero).

In this case, an individual is in a gambling position. He or she can accept the gamble, by not consuming the prevention good, or can opt out of the gamble by consuming it, thereby ensuring avoidance of the outcome. Opting out, however, is not costless as the prevention good can be consumed only at some cost; monetary or in terms of time, etc.

A person can be defined as being risk neutral if he or she is indifferent between the certainty of a loss X (in this case the cost of the good) and any gamble with expected outcome X (in this case the present value of the expected loss). A risk averse person will, by definition (Kahneman and Tversky 1979), always prefer the certainty to the gamble—that is, he or she will always consume the good when its cost is just equal to the present value of the expected loss. The more risk averse the individual is, the greater the cost he or she will be prepared to incur to avoid the gamble (consume the good).

9.6.6. *The demand for prevention goods*

Figure 9.1 represents the economic principle that demand depends on the interaction of the utility yielded by a good and its cost. Conventionally, the term 'price' is used rather than cost, as for most economic goods the money price represents the cost to the consumer. As explained earlier, however, the money price of many prevention goods may not be the prime element of cost to the consumer, and costs such as forgone work and leisure time, or pain and inconvenience, may be the prime cost elements.

The above economic principles, as a part of what we can now call the 'Utility Model of Preventive Behaviour' have many policy implications.

9.7. Policy implication of the utility model

Prevention is seen by many as the key to improving the health of populations. If it is agreed that more prevention is a good thing, then in terms of the utility model, what is being sought is an increase in the demand for prevention goods and, of course, a decrease in the demand for hazard goods.

Many definitions of prevention abound, and there are many conflicting views about what the objectives of a prevention policy should be. The above-stated aim is by no means universally accepted. For a start, the definition of a prevention good used in the model conflicts with the views of many working in the area of health education who consider health education itself to be a prevention good (Cohen 1984a). In their view a successful health education campaign is one where the message is received by a large number of people. A

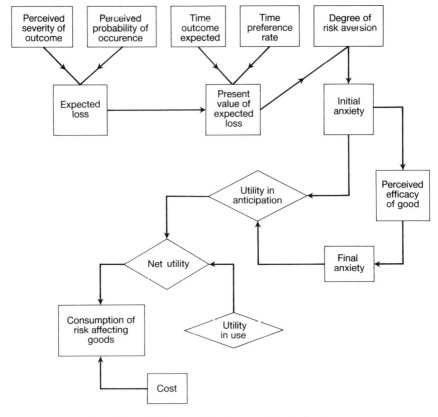

Fig. 9.1   Utility model of preventive behaviour.

message, however, does not of itself reduce risk unless it elicits the appropriate behaviour change. Any campaigns which get a message across, or even change attitudes will not be 'prevention' under our model's definition.

Figure 9.1 shows that preventive behaviour can be influenced by measures affecting perceptions of (1) cost, (2) utility-in-anticipation, and (3) utility-in-use. The most *cost-effective* measure or combination of measures will be that which produces the greatest change in the quantity of a prevention good consumed for any given expenditure.

The utility model suggests that an examination of both the nature of the good affecting risk, and the target audience ought to provide insights into the most cost-effective approach. This has the advantage over the household production models, reviewed earlier, in that its concentration is on the demand for individual prevention and hazards goods rather than a more general 'desire to be healthy'. It has an advantage over the psychological models in that it recognizes the importance of such economic concepts as discounting and the basic cost versus benefit framework.

9.7.1. *Factors affecting utility-in-anticipation*

Figure 9.1 shows that the level of utility-in-anticipation is affected by:

—the perceived effectiveness of the prevention good;
—the perceived severity of the outcome;
—the level of initial anxiety associated with the outcome;
—the perceived probability of the outcome occurring;
—the degree of risk aversion;
—the length of time before the outcome is anticipated;
—the individual's personal time preference rate.

The first point to note is that the provision of information that changes perceptions can alter any of the above *except* for the degree of risk aversion and the time preference rate. Any attempt to change these last two are clearly an attempt to impose one preferred set of values over another.

If a policy wishes to avoid adopting such an elitist approach then a close examination of the target audience is needed. Groups that can be shown to have a relatively high rate of time preference or a relatively low degree of risk aversion will have lower levels of initial anxiety than will groups with the opposite characteristics. In these cases the effectiveness of health education campaigns aimed at increasing perceptions of the relatively less important utility-in-anticipation will be lower, other things being equal, than campaigns aimed at groups with the opposite characteristics. In such cases, attempts to alter utility-in-use (see below), or measures to reduce cost, may prove to be more cost-effective than conventional health education aimed essentially at utility-in-anticipation.

9.7.2. *Factors affecting utility-in-use*

Utility-in-use is what is normally conveyed by the simple term 'utility' in conventional economic analysis, and conventional advertising is the normal means of increasing perceptions of utility in order to increase demand. Though it may seem rather obvious that singing the virtues of the fun/pleasure/ enjoyment aspects of a good can increase the demand for it, the utility model emphasizes that this conventional demand manipulator will be more important, the greater is the amount of utility-in-use relative to utility-in-anticipation provided by the good.

Cohen and Mooney (1985) developed a taxonomy of prevention goods and hazard goods, which categorizes such goods as 'wholly preventive', 'partly preventive', 'ordinary', 'partly hazardous', or 'wholly hazardous', according to the relative amounts of utility-in-use (positive or negative) and utility-in-anticipation (again positive or negative) which they yield. The greater is the proportion of utility-in-use, the more effective will normal advertising be as a means of manipulating demand.

For example, a cigarette is a hazard good which provides obvious utility-in-use to smokers but also negative utility-in-anticipation from the knowledge that smoking increases the risks of lung cancer, heart disease, bronchitis, etc. If the positive utility-in-use from smoking greatly overshadows the negative utility-in-anticipation for most smokers, then an anti-smoking campaign aimed at reducing perceptions of utility-in-use, perhaps by emphasizing the annoyance caused to non-smokers, may prove a more efficient way of reducing smoking than a campaign that tries to increase perceptions of (dis)utility-in-anticipation via the health message.

9.7.3. Factors affecting cost

Ultimately, the decision to consume a good will be based *inter alia* on a comparison of utility and cost. If the objective of prevention policy is to increase the demand for prevention goods and reduce the demand for hazard goods, (although we realize that many health educationists may dispute this aim), then measures aimed at reducing the cost side of the equation may prove to be more cost-effective than either form of utility manipulation.

9.8. The role of health education in influencing the demand for prevention

If, as has just been claimed, health education is not prevention *per se*, then what is it? In terms of the Grossman type models it could be viewed as the information which individuals require to enable them to make efficient consumption choices. But if this were all that health education is, there could be no justification in, for example, trying to influence people's values, or their degrees of risk aversion, or their personal time preference rates. Clearly much health education (defined as the output of health education organizations) contains this type of message.

9.8.1. What is health education?

Health education is a major policy tool in the pursuit of prevention. An interesting feature of health education is that there seems to be little agreement on precisely what it is. In 1981, Edinburgh hosted the First International Conference on Health Education and the Media. In his *British Medical Journal* review of the congress, Smith (1981) stated that 'an outsider might expect health educators, who have been around for many years, to be agreed on what they were trying to do, but this was not so'.

Economists do not claim to have the final answer, but the economic perspective does at least provide one concise definition which is consistent with this particular way of looking at the subject.

Health Education attempts to alter the demand for prevention goods and hazard goods using information and guidance which highlights the benefits of reducing the risks of illness or injury. (Cohen 1983, p. 56)

This definition is firmly tied to the 'behaviour' part of the changed awareness, changed attitudes, changed behaviour continuum. If the view is held that health education itself is a consumption good, then health education programmes will be evaluated in terms of whether or not the message is received. If attitude change is perceived to be the key, then programmes will be evaluated in terms consistent with that objective.

By the definition used here, neither knowledge nor attitude changes will affect risk unless they elicit the appropriate behaviour change. Neither can therefore be viewed as objectives of health education within this definition.

This does not mean that there can be no benefits associated with making people more aware and knowledgeable. Far from it. But often expenditures on health education are drawn from wider health budgets, as is the case with District Health Authorities in the UK. In these cases the opportunity costs are in terms of health forgone from alternative health programmes. It is not unreasonable to focus on the health output of health education and to argue that programmes whose objectives do not go beyond education should not be seen as alternatives to expenditures on health care or other forms of prevention. They should not be included in the definition of health education used when such common-output, inter-programme comparisons are made.

Furthermore, the definition used here is inconsistent with the notion that anything done by health educationists is health education. An anti-smoking campaign that tries to reduce utility-in-use by making smokers feel like social pariahs is not health education by this definition. Similarly, an advertising campaign by the maker of high-fibre breakfast cereal which highlights the preventive benefits of dietary fibre, is health education.

The advantages of looking at health education in this way are threefold. First, as stated above, it is consistent with the aim of maximizing health benefits from limited resources. Second, the criteria for programme appraisal are specified because the aim of health education is explicit. Finally, the focus on risk changes is consistent with the fact that both the incidence of illness and the effectiveness of most forms of prevention are matters of probability.

9.9. Conclusion

This chapter has shown that an analysis of the demand for prevention involves more than may at first meet the eye. It is difficult to pursue any such analysis without a clear understanding of precisely what the expression 'prevention' means. Agreement on this has been long awaited.

Theoretical models are of value in that a better understanding of the factors that determine the demand for prevention provides messages for public policy, but the value of the message is only as good as the value of the analysis upon which it rests. If important features of prevention are omitted, such as the idea that individuals can receive peace of mind from the knowledge that their risk levels have been reduced, then important implications for policy can be missed. It is to policy that we now turn.

10 Towards a prevention strategy

10.1. Introduction

For over a decade there have been explicit policy statements calling for a shift of emphasis away from treatment and cure and toward prevention as part of a new health strategy. Both the UK and the US governments, for example, have espoused an overall, comprehensive prevention policy as the way forward in trying to reduce morbidity and mortality (Department of Health and Social Security 1977; Department of Health, Education, and Welfare 1980). With so much having been said, it is reasonable to ask why more hasn't been done.

One reason why prevention has not made the advances that some might have hoped for is that it covers such a wide spectrum of outcomes and risk factors. Responsibility is thus spread over a wide variety of different actors. Those who take decisions on running health screening programmes are unlikely to communicate with those who take decisions about environmental health. Neither are likely to be familiar with the activities of the charity which seeks to prevent alcohol and drug abuse. In turn, those who run the charity will probably know little about the government department responsible for running anti-smoking campaigns. The government department responsible for advice about healthy diets may not communicate on this issue with the department that subsidizes the production of food, some of which may be bad for health.

There is, of course, no reason why any should be concerned about what the others are doing as each has a specific remit to deal with a specific problem. However, Chapter 1 has shown that all can be viewed as producing a similar output regardless of the particular risk factors or preventable outcomes each addresses. An overall prevention policy is about getting as much of this common output as is possible given the resource constraint.

The need for choice is inescapable in prevention policy. The resources available for prevention will always be scarce relative to the demands made on them, and Chapters 4 to 7 have shown that while there can be no single best way of making these choices, economic efficiency is one important criterion for choice. Prevention programmes with the same resource costs but different levels of output (benefits) are not equally efficient. If we simplify and argue for the moment that prevention is about saving life-years, and if it is further

133

assumed that saving a life-year by preventing a road traffic fatality has the same value as saving a life-year by preventing a heart attack then, other things being equal, the programme with the lowest cost per life-year saved is the most efficient and should be pursued most vigorously. The fact that the two programmes may be run by different organizations and aimed at different risk factors does not matter in the pursuit of efficiency.

We have argued for some time (Cohen and Henderson 1983) that an effective and efficient prevention policy needs an integrated strategy, directed by a 'Minister for Prevention'. In the UK, the NHS reforms, with their separation of hospitals as providers of care from District Health Authorities whose job is to assess their residents' health needs, offer new opportunities to pursue local prevention strategies. In addition, the English Department of Health has proposed to set targets for improving the health of the nation (Department of Health 1991) taking into account the role to be played by other ministries. Thus, some positive steps have been taken towards the more coordinated approach represented by the idea of a Minister for Prevention.

This chapter examines what information base a Minister for Prevention would require to plan a prevention strategy, and how on the basis of that information he or she should plan prevention policy. The first section indicates the potential for prevention on different diseases and problems. The next section explores how current resources for prevention are being used in the US and the UK. A 'Prevention Programme Budget' for the UK is then presented to illustrate the feasibility and the value of the programme budgeting approach. This is followed by a discussion of how such information can be of value, and what additional information and considerations will be needed in the pursuit of overall efficiency.

10.2. What can be gained through prevention?

Figures 10.1 and 10.2 show the potential years of life lost by major causes for the UK and Canada. Such information, coupled with information on the extent to which each cause of death is preventable—and the cost of prevention at the margin—is clearly necessary for a coherent prevention strategy. For example, a Canadian Minister for Prevention may wish to analyse more carefully the marginal costs of reducing 'non-medical' deaths (motor vehicle accidents, other accidents, and suicide) which represented three of the four largest causes of potential years of life lost in Canada. In Britain the focus may be elsewhere, as such non-medical deaths represent a relatively small number of preventable years of life lost in the UK compared with other causes.

Gaining life-years is not the only objective of prevention. Prevention seeks to alter the health profile shown in Figure 1.1; extending it to the north (better health) and east (longer life) of the graph. The benefits of such profile changes

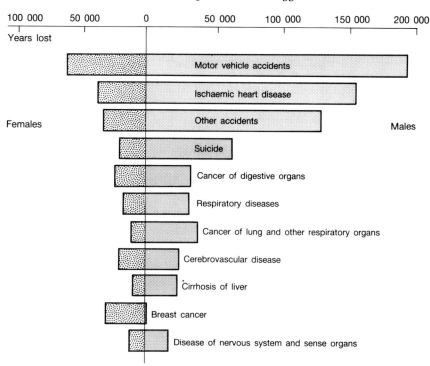

Fig. 10.1 Distribution of potential years of life lost between ages 1 and 70 by major causes, by sex (Canada 1974). *Source*: Romeder and McWhinnie 1977.

fall under several categories. As was shown in Chapters 5 and 6, more health can mean the saving of resources and improvements in productivity. In addition, there is the value attached to health *per se*.

Prevention is not only capable of producing more health, but can also, as was shown in Chapter 9, provide utility-in-anticipation from the knowledge that individuals are less at risk of illness or injury if they engage in prevention. Moreover, many preventive measures confer other benefits, such as lower risk of fires with reduced smoking and less violence and other social problems with reduced alcohol consumption.

A prevention strategy should consider all of these when examining what can be gained through prevention, and a full economic evaluation of prevention should account for all. However, it is likely that there will be particular interest in the scope for reducing health service costs and reducing the output loss to industry from preventable illness and injury as these represent high profile and politically sensitive issues which tend to be

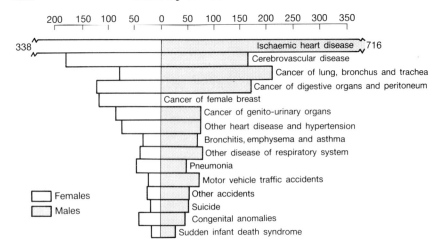

Fig. 10.2 Potential years of life lost between 0 and 90 by major causes, by sex, in England and Wales 1985 (rates per 10 000 population). *Source*: Office of Population Censuses and Surveys 1987.

prominent in priority documents. Accordingly, the next sections deal with these two areas.

10.2.1. *The potential for saving health care resources*

The costs of treating illnesses and injuries that can be reduced through prevention are sizeable. Table 10.1 illustrates the health care costs imposed by some of these.

It would be misleading to use the term 'preventable costs' for these figures, as that would imply that they could be avoided in their entirety. Clearly this is not the case. Such labelling would further imply that outcomes with the highest costs should be pursued most vigorously. This is equally false. What is important is their responsiveness to prevention. The fact that a disease happens to impose a high resource cost on the health service is irrelevant if little can be done via prevention to reduce it.

While the ultimate objective of prevention is a reduction in morbidity and mortality, the time delay between the prevention and the fall in morbidity and mortality often means that operational objectives are in 'intermediate' terms. Thus it is more common to find the objective of an immunization campaign to be in terms of increasing vaccine uptake rates rather than in falls in the incidence of the disease. The aims of anti-smoking campaigns will be expressed in terms of reduced smoking prevalence rather than the incidence of smoking-related diseases. The assumption, of course, is that success in the intermediate objective will lead to success in the final objective.

Table 10.1 Health care costs of various illnesses and injuries, UK 1980–1981 (£ Millions)

Lung cancer	39.3
Bladder cancer	13.3
Chronic bronchitis and emphysema	55.2
Ischaemic heart disease	142.2
Occupational accidents and diseases	78.0
Dental diseases	406.0
Road traffic accidents	69·0

Source: derived from Cohen and Henderson 1983

This can cause problems when assessing the effect of prevention on health care costs. Increasing vaccine uptake rates will affect health care costs differently, according to the risk level of the target group. Reducing smoking prevalence will affect health care costs differently according to the age, sex, and smoking characteristics of those who give up. So how might the economic benefits of reduced smoking prevalence be estimated?

Table 10.2 shows how the cost to the UK National Health Service can be broken down by age and sex for five major smoking-related diseases. Not surprisingly, the majority of these costs are in the older age groups—although the illness which manifests itself in later years is inevitably the consequence of smoking behaviour over many previous years.

Since many anti-smoking efforts are aimed specifically at keeping young people from taking up smoking, Cohen (1984b) estimated the effect which a non-smoking generation would have on health care costs over time. On the assumption that no one currently aged under 16 takes up smoking, but those currently over 16 continue to smoke as before, costs of smoking to the NHS will look like those in Figure 10.3.

It is interesting that since most costs occur in the older age groups, total costs do not fall significantly for many years. Indeed, as far ahead as the year 2020 the cost to the NHS with a non-smoking generation will have fallen by only 7 per cent from the 1980 figure (£157 million).

The actual saving owing to the non-smoking generation is greater than this, however, owing to a different population age structure in 2020. The 60 + age group, in which most smoking morbidity occurs will be some 17 per cent larger in 2020 than 1980. This is independent of the non-smoking generation who will not have reached that age by then. Accordingly, cost to the NHS for this older age group will rise considerably, and the 7 per cent fall in total costs

Table 10.2　Costs to the NHS of diseases attributable to smoking by cause and age, England and Wales 1981 (£ millions)

Cause	Males aged					All males
	16–24	25–34	35–49	50–59	60+	
Lung cancer	0	0	0.6	12.4	26.0	39.0
Bladder cancer	0	0.2	0.1	0.5	4.5	5.3
Ischaemic heart disease	0	0	1.7	5.3	14.1	21.1
Chronic bronchitis/emphysema	0	0	1.2	7.8	31.7	40.7
Peptic ulcer	0.3	0.6	1.5	1.7	4.8	8.9
All	0.3	0.8	5.1	27.7	81.1	115.0

Cause	Females aged					All females
	16–24	25–34	35–49	50–59	60+	
Lung cancer	0.9	0.9	1.0	1.4	4.3	8.5
Bladder cancer	0	0	0.2	0.1	1.2	1.4
Ischaemic heart disease	0	0.1	1.3	5.6	7.8	14.8
Chronic bronchitis/emphysema	0	0	1.2	6.2	7.7	15.2
Peptic ulcer	0.1	0.3	0.7	0.3	1.5	2.9
All	1.0	1.3	4.4	13.5	22.5	42.8

Total all persons = 157.8

Source: Cohen 1984b

from the 1980 figure due to the non-smoking generation will in fact represent a 21 per cent reduction in what the 2020 cost would otherwise be (£185.9 million). Such data are clearly relevant when devising policies to consider how different types of prevention programmes can affect health care costs.

In the US, Oster, Colditz, and Kelly (1984) have not only broken down the health care costs of treating smoking-related diseases by age and sex, but have also taken into account smoking behaviour. The lifetime savings in health care costs which can be realized by people of various ages and smoking habits giving up the habit are shown in Table 10.3.

Note that the health service benefits owing to reduced risk of lung cancer are greater than those for reduced risk of coronary heart disease (CHD) even though heart disease imposes a greater health care burden than lung cancer

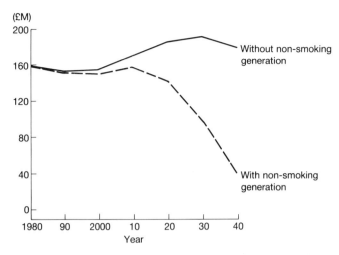

Fig. 10.3 Cost of smoking to the NHS (1980–2040). *Source*: Cohen 1984.

(see Table 10.1). The fact that lung cancer costs can be reduced by a greater amount via prevention than CHD costs is what matters. More estimates along these lines are necessary if prevention policy is to be coherent and rationally based.

10.2.2. *The potential for preventing productivity losses*

The economic burden of injury and illness represented by lost productive output often overshadows health care costs. Prevention of illness and injury increases the flow of healthy days which in turn increases productive capacity. Although non-remunerated output is also a benefit from increased healthy days, productivity that contributes to Gross National Product will inevitably be looked upon with more interest than productivity improvements in the non-working population by those wishing to be re-elected.

Table 10.4 shows the estimated value of output lost caused by smoking, alcohol abuse, road traffic accidents, and occupational accidents and diseases in the UK for 1980–1981. In all cases the value of the output lost is approximately ten times the value of the health service resource costs. From the prevention point of view these potential benefits will be dependent on the ages and other characteristics of those at whom prevention is aimed.

Table 10.5 shows how total sickness absence owing to smoking-related diseases for 1980, in the UK, can be divided by age and sex.

If the non-smoking generation discussed above were to become a reality, the costs of sickness absence in the UK over time would look like their depiction in Figure 10.4.

Table 10.3 Health care benefits of quitting smoking due to reductions in risks of lung cancer, coronary heart disease, and chronic obstructive pulmonary disease by age, sex, and smoking characteristics

	Lung cancer		CHD		COPD	
	Light	Heavy	Light	Heavy	Light	Heavy
Men aged						
30–34	526	1113	NA	NA	NA	NA
35–39	597	1233	211	727	267	1030
40–44	657	1318	200	602	291	1123
45–49	698	1346	162	425	307	1186
50–54	709	1295	112	240	317	1222
55–59	674	1142	52	89	320	1237
60–64	578	901	9	17	322	1241
65–69	438	632	0	0	305	1172
70–74	292	395	0	0	267	1021
75–79	174	226	0	0	212	808
Women aged						
30–34	192	581	NA	NA	NA	NA
35–39	214	637	35a	167a	186	986
40–44	233	677	34a	125a	208	1099
45–49	246	695	62	195	227	1203
50–54	251	678	49	124	246	1301
55–59	241	597	23	48	266	1407
60–64	201	460	5	9	290	1537
65–69	145	318	0	0	287	1513
70–74	97	206	0	0	250	1314
75–79	63	126	0	0	196	1024

Note: 1980 dollars per smoker, discounted at 3 per cent annual rate, assume 1 per cent productivity growth.
Light smoker 1–14 cigarettes per day. Heavy smoker > 35 per day
a = for myocardial infarction only.
Source: Oster, Colditz, and Kelly 1984

The cost of sickness absence in terms of lost output will rise dramatically if smoking continues as at present owing to demographic changes, and allowing for a modest 1 per cent growth in productivity over time. With a non-smoking generation the effect will be negligible until the year 2000, but after 2010 will be dramatic.

Table 10.4 Value of output lost due to various causes, UK 1980–81 (£ millions)

Cause	Lost output
Smoking	1471
Alcohol abuse	774
Road traffic accidents	679
Occupational accidents and diseases	764

Source: Cohen and Henderson 1983

Table 10.5 Sickness absence by age and cause due to smoking (days, thousands) GB 1980, and cost of sickness absence

Cause	Days lost by males aged				
	16–24	25–34	35–49	50–59	60+
Lung cancer	0	0	0	58.1	57·8
Bladder cancer	0.3	1.0	0.8	2.0	15.8
Ischaemic heart disease	1.6	2.8	558.0	1814.8	2535.1
Chronic bronchitis/ emphysema	1.5	14.5	486.9	3013.5	5816.0
Peptic ulcer	55.4	128.7	309.3	288.2	188.4

	Days lost by females aged				
	16–24	25–34	35–49	50–59	60+
Lung cancer	0	0	0	0	0
Bladder cancer	0	0.3	0.7	0	4.1
Ischaemic heart disease	0.2	2.3	34.7	152.9	22.3
Chronic bronchitis/ emphysema	0.3	2.6	45.8	235.3	31.5
Peptic ulcer	4.0	12.2	23.4	10.5	5.6

Total days lost 15 939.2
Total cost of sickness absence due to smoking = £611.2 million
Note: figures represent estimated days lost *to smoking* by cause, not total days lost by cause
Source: Cohen 1984b

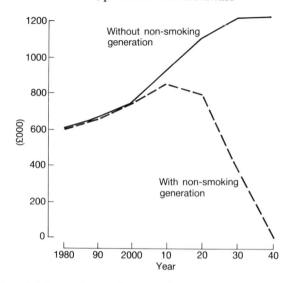

Fig. 10.4.   Cost of sickness absence due to smoking with and without a non-smoking
generation (1980–2040). *Source*: Cohen 1984.

In the US, Oster, Colditz, and Kelly (1984) have also estimated the lifetime
benefits of increased labour output for different age groups and different
smoking habits as shown in Table 10.6. They explicitly included the value of
increased housework. Note that in all cases the output benefits exceed the
health care gains for the younger age groups.

During periods of full employment there are few problems in estimating the
value of the extra output resulting from an increase in healthy days. When
unemployment persists, however, it is necessary to estimate what proportion
of increased healthy time is likely to result in increased marketed output. At the
extreme one could take the stance adopted by Williams (1985) who in his
study of the economics of coronary artery bypass grafting, stated 'Given the
amount of unemployment which is expected to persist in the near future,
increases in productivity that might be associated with employment gains
have been disregarded' (p. 326). Given the uncertainty regarding the future of
the national economy and the probability of being unemployed, the issue of
productivity benefits from prevention is inevitably a difficult one.

10.3. Who spends what on prevention?

In order to direct incremental prevention resources to their most cost-effective
uses and to determine whether marginal shifts of existing resources could

Table 10.6 Productivity benefits of quitting smoking due to reductions in risks of lung cancer, coronary heart disease, and chronic obstructive pulmonary disease by age, sex, and smoking characteristics

	Lung cancer		CHD		COPD	
	Light	Heavy	Light	Heavy	Light	Heavy
Men aged						
30–34	2896	5685	NA	NA	NA	NA
35–39	2824	5189	2120	7818	6616	25861
40–44	2462	4161	1709	5214	5741	22678
45–49	1848	2886	1077	2764	4281	16083
50–54	1183	1748	546	1109	2693	10129
55–59	669	967	174	298	1420	5359
60–64	363	509	20	39	738	2799
65–69	191	258	0	0	434	1651
70–74	95	123	0	0	255	969
75–79	44	55	0	0	151	573
Women aged						
30–34	617	1768	NA	NA	NA	NA
35–39	604	1643	152a	788a	1812	9373
40–44	543	1408	130a	454a	1681	8701
45–49	450	1119	162	534	1436	7442
50–54	347	825	95	233	1137	5904
55–59	248	537	37	75	889	4627
60–64	146	288	5	11	732	3821
65–69	68	129	0	0	505	2632
70–74	27	52	0	0	274	1428
75–79	11	21	0	0	135	700

Note: 1980 dollars per smoker, discounted at 3 per cent annual rate, assume 1 per cent productivity growth.
Light smoker 1–14 cigarettes per day. Heavy smoker > 35 per day
a = for myocardial infarction only.
Source: Oster, Colditz and Kelly 1984

improve overall efficiency, it is necessary to have some idea of what is currently being spent on prevention and by whom. Ideally such information is required on expenditures in private markets as well as by public bodies.

Many prevention and all hazard goods are produced by firms operating in private markets. We saw in Chapter 3 that *perfect* markets will be self-regulating, thus obviating any need for government intervention, and the arguments for government intervention in the case of *imperfect* markets are the same for prevention or hazard goods as for any other types of goods. There is, however, a great deal of prevention provided by the public sector and by charitable and voluntary organizations. In these cases the absence of a price mechanism and the signals which prices give to suppliers and consumers in free markets, suggests that policy makers will wish to concentrate attention on the prevention resource deployment in this sector of the economy. Moreover, these are the resources over which the Minister would have the most direct control. In the following two sections we examine the deployment of prevention resources by public and charitable bodies in the US and the UK.

10.3.1. *Who spends what on prevention in the United States?*

Regan (1986) has identified federally funded preventive health programmes in the US. Table 10.7 shows the 1984 'budget obligations' (which may be read as a proxy for expenditure) of four programmes within the Department of Health and Human Services.

An immediate problem is that, apart from 'Preventive health and health services' which is purely preventive, the figures represent total budgets including expenditure on non-preventive activities. This is acknowledged, but because the preventive activities of each budget are not identified as such, there is no attempt to determine the prevention proportion of each.

The same problem occurs with other activities which are only 'minimally' preventive. For example, Regan describes the preventive activities carried out under Medicare (total federal outlay for 1984 = $57.5 billion) and Medicaid ($20.1 billion), but because of the accounting methods used does not attempt to estimate what the expenditure on these preventive activities might be.

Table 10.7   Budget obligations for Department of Health and Human Services block grants, fiscal year 1984

Block	Budget ($ thousands)
Alcohol, drug abuse, and mental health	462 000
Primary care	536 442
Maternal and child health	398 964
Preventive health and health services	88 187

Source: Regan 1986

This is a general problem that bedevils any attempt to estimate what is currently being spent on prevention. Until such time as better accounting allows for the separation of the prevention expenditures of those bodies whose activities are not wholly prevention orientated, roundabout methods will have to be used to estimate what is currently being spent.

Table 10.8 shows the 'budget obligations' for preventive programmes run by other federal agencies for 1984. Here the categories are more specifically preventive, although not all budgets should be regarded as wholly for prevention. For example, 'The National Institute of Occupational Safety and Health . . . is involved in extensive research on causes of *and cures for* occupational diseases' (p. 124, emphasis ours). The $65.8 million is thus an overstatement of expenditure on prevention.

Another major problem lies in deciding where to draw the line regarding what should be included. Regan identifies $16.9 billion 'budget obligations' for the Food and Nutrition Service Programs of the US Department of Agriculture, but acknowledges that 'Although these nutrition services are not necessarily preventive in each case, some of the recipients would not have a nutritionally sound diet without them' (p. 126).

The point is valid, but by the same logic it could be argued that expenditures to replace damp, dangerous, and overcrowded housing should be included as prevention expenditures. Certainly, the effects of better housing on health are recognized, but expenditure on better housing is not primarily for preventive reasons. Similarly, no one would deny the preventive aspects of refuse collection, but even if garbage were not a health hazard it would still be collected. It would thus be almost impossible to try to estimate the proportion of expenditure on housing or refuse collection that is preventive, and despite Regan's observation on the preventive aspects of better nutrition, it would probably be more realistic to limit discussion to those activities that are more explicitly preventive.

The total 'budget obligation' of Tables 10.7 and 10.8 is $22.5 billion. This figure is not intended to represent an estimate of total expenditure on prevention in the US. As Regan states 'The preventive programs outlined here are not a complete index of federally funded preventive health services . . . (It) does provide, however, a broad overview of the types of agencies and programs involved in disease prevention and health promotion' (p. 121). It is thus consistent with the methodology arguments of Section 4.2.

10.3.2. *Who spends what on prevention in the United Kingdom?*

In 1983, and in the light of all the policy statements that had been made in the UK concerning the importance of shifting the emphasis of health policy from treatment to prevention, the current authors attempted to determine what

Table 10.8   Budget obligations for various federal agencies
and programs, fiscal year 1984

Agency/Program	Budget obligation ($ thousands)
Centres for Disease Control	
Sexually transmitted diseases	54 688
Infectious disease prevention	51 633
Epidemic services	47 554
Immunizations	42 068
Chronic and environmental disease prevention	25 953
Occupational Safety and Health (NIOSH)	65 872
Occupational Safety and Health Administration	
Safety and health standards	5 910
Federal enforcement	84 807
State enforcement	49 620
Compliance assistance	35 857
Mine Safety and Health Administration	
Enforcement (coal)	76 220
Enforcement (metal–non-metal)	29 056
Enforcement (standards development)	886
Assessments	2 031
Educational policy and development	11 923
Environmental Protection Agency	
Air quality	113 280
Water quality	114 086
Drinking water	40 189
Hazardous waste	67 884
Pesticides	21 344
Toxic substances	23 355
Radiation	2 974
National Highway Traffic Safety Administration	
All safety	106 000

Source: Regan 1986

was then being spent on prevention, by whom, and for what (Cohen and
Henderson 1983).

The *raison d'être* for the exercise was the recognition of fragmented
responsibility for prevention in the UK, and the perceived need for coordination. It was felt that existing prevention 'policy' was ineffective and that

some form of organization and control was an essential step in making prevention policy work.

In order to provide information on who was doing what in prevention, three principal areas were identified:

(1) the NHS;
(2) non-NHS public sector;
(3) charitable and voluntary organizations.

Two points made in Section 10.3.1 should be stressed again. First, the choice of what is to be considered prevention is inevitably somewhat arbitrary. Expenditures on such things as improved housing and refuse collection undoubtedly have a preventive element, but as they would be undertaken even if they were not partly preventive they have not been included in this exercise. Second, it is not possible to be wholly comprehensive. It is inevitable that some organizations, especially those operating at local level will be overlooked. In addition, there is much prevention carried out by industry that would be difficult to determine in an exercise of this type and all prevention carried out by private individuals cannot be dealt with here. Therefore, as was stated earlier in the case of the US, the total *identified* expenditure on prevention should be viewed as just that, and not as an estimate of total expenditure.

10.3.2.1. *Preventive expenditure within the NHS* A major difficulty in assessing the expenditure on prevention within a formal health sector arises in trying to separate tertiary prevention from treatment. Most services in the NHS play a tertiary preventive role to such an extent that the Department of Health and Social Security has stated that 'a meaningful estimate of the total sum spent on prevention cannot be achieved, and that to attempt to do so would throw the emphasis on certain services at the expense of others with a less apparent concern for prevention' (Department of Health and Social Security 1977). The analysis that follows is therefore restricted to expenditures on primary and secondary prevention, for reasons purely of data limitations.

The top part of Table 10.9 shows the estimated prevention expenditures for Family Practitioner Services, both medical and dental, Community Health Services, and Hospital Services. For General Medical Services, it was assumed that all services directed at otherwise healthy people (vaccination, sterilization, contraceptive advice, and health education) are primary prevention. Medical examinations for reasons other than illness—that is, non-symptomatic examinations—are considered a form of screening in this exercise. Also classed as screening are cervical cytology, and all pre- and post-natal care for normal pregnancy.

In the case of General Dental Services, expenditure on prevention was determined using three expenditure classifications of the Dental Estimates Boards; examination of normal teeth, scaling and gum treatment, and removal of calculus. Community Health Service estimates excluded domiciliary treatments as these were deemed as either care, cure, or tertiary prevention. All other community services, including school health services, both medical and dental, health visiting, family planning, health education, and fluoridation, were classed as primary or secondary prevention.

Preventive expenditure in the hospital sector is based solely on maternity out-patient expenditure as this was the only major service which could be identified as being preventive and for which data were available. Clearly services such as sterilization are also preventive, but such services are not costed separately.

Table 10.9 shows total prevention expenditure within the NHS to be around £550 million, or nearly 6 per cent of a total of £9472 million for these services

Table 10.9   Expenditure on prevention in the UK 1980–1981 (£ thousands)

National Health Service	
Family Practitioner Services:	
General Medical Services	75 978
General Dental Services	101 533
Community Health Services	312 652
Hospital Services	59 385
Total	549 548
Non-NHS public sector:	
Ministry of Agriculture, Fisheries and Food	34
Department of Employment (Health and safety at work)	72 167
Department of the Environment	268
Department of Health and Social Security/ Scottish Home and Health Department	19 882
Home Office	45
Northern Ireland Office	109
Scottish Office	1
Department of Trade	30
Central Office of Information	100
Local Authorities (Environmental health)	309 000
Total	401 636
Private and Voluntary Organizations	
Total for 19 identified bodies	15 500
Total identified UK expenditure on prevention	966 684

Source: Cohen and Henderson 1983

in 1981. (Total expenditure on the NHS, gross of all charges, for 1980–1981 was £11 825 million.)

10.3.2.2. *Prevention expenditure in the non-NHS public sector*   Under this heading all expenditures not explicitly undertaken for preventive reasons have been excluded even if they have an indirect effect on future ill-health. Thus, for example, expenditures of the four UK Sports Councils (£26 million in 1980–1981) have been omitted even though the effect of exercise on health is recognized. It is clear that the Sports Councils exist to promote sport for its own sake.

The expenditures of thirty-two bodies were identified. Of these, twenty-six were wholly preventive, and estimates had to be made of the preventive proportion of the remaining six. On this basis, a total prevention expenditure of just over £400 million was identified.

10.3.2.3. *Prevention expenditure by charitable and voluntary organizations*   As government is not the only source of preventive activities, a Minister for Prevention would also clearly be interested in the nature and extent of prevention outside the public sector. In this exercise, £15.5 million of preventive expenditure by nineteen private and voluntary organizations was derived, based primarily on a survey carried out in 1981 (Cohen and Moir 1981). Under this heading in particular it is important to stress that the identified expenditure is not an estimate of the true total.

Though classed as charitable or voluntary, the extent of public money involved is considerable. Fifteen of the nineteen bodies received grants from the Department of Health and Social Security and grants from other government departments were sizeable. Though officially independent of government control, these organizations are heavily supported by government finance and the public monies channelled into the private and voluntary agencies ought to be employed in the most efficient way.

10.4. A prevention programme budget

While the identified expenditure in the previous section is not intended to represent the total of all expenditures which have an effect on levels of risk, it can be of assistance in identifying at least some of the resources available for prevention, and hence potentially the responsibility of a Minister for Prevention. Government plays a major role in prevention both directly through the NHS and other public bodies, and through the funding of charitable and voluntary organizations. A Prevention Minister will thus have direct control over much expenditure, but will also have as part of his or her remit responsibility for encouraging the private sector to take more cognizance of prevention.

Figure 10.5 shows how the identified expenditure of £967 million is divided into eleven programmes of prevention. Presentation of the data in this format allows consideration of whether the balance between programmes is as desired and will focus attention on broad objectives and priorities. Moreover, since every decision to alter the balance will involve changes in costs and benefits at the margins, the approach forces consideration on benefit valuation, even if it cannot be done explicitly as part of the exercise. A Prevention Minister will be forced to speculate on what will have to be sacrificed compared with what will be gained by any changes in relative programme size. This approach ought to lead to a more rational prevention strategy than would result from a focus on individual prevention programmes.

It should be noted that as this approach is not evaluative (see Section 4.2) no policy conclusions can be drawn directly from it. The proportions of total expenditure shown in Figure 10.5 do not in themselves indicate any need for change. However, presentation of the data in this format can raise many questions thereby suggesting where further investigation ought to be directed.

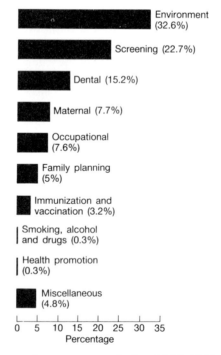

Fig. 10.5 The UK prevention programme budget 1980–1981. *Source*: Cohen and Henderson 1984a.

Repeating this exercise for earlier and subsequent years would show changes in the relative importance of the different programmes over time as well as allow projection into the future. Much could be gleaned from such an exercise, particularly if changes in expenditure could be compared with measures on the output side (i.e. reduced morbidity and mortality).

10.5. Discussion

After seven chapters of micro-analysis this chapter has returned to the wider view. Understanding micro issues such as consumer behaviour, the operations of markets, and the assessment of individual prevention initiatives is vital, but will not lead to greater prevention unless there is some means of channelling this into a broad strategy. This chapter has tried to show that an efficient strategy can be devised, but there is clearly a long way to go.

A principal message to emerge here is the vital role that relevant information plays in the devising of efficient strategies. Related to this is the notion that information on its own is not enough. Mechanisms are needed to ensure that responsibility for prevention is not so fragmented that identified efficiencies cannot be exploited because of the absence of channels of communication or the presence of in-built obstacles to efficiency.

11 Prevention: the contribution of health economics

11.1. Introduction

This book has attempted to show that there is much that economics can offer to the analysis of prevention. The contribution of economics can be grouped under seven broad headings:

(1) the effect of prevention on the economy;
(2) the role of economic policy as part of prevention policy;
(3) the role of government in the pursuit of prevention;
(4) the appraisal of prevention;
(5) the provision of information to assist policy making;
(6) an understanding of preventive behaviour;
(7) a framework for the setting and implementation of prevention policy.

A prerequisite to all of the above is a clear understanding of precisely what is being discussed, and one of the first objectives of this book was to ensure that economists working in the area of prevention should not be subject to the sort of criticism levelled at health educators by Smith (1981). It will be recalled (see quote on p. 130) that Smith found an absence of agreement among health educators who attended an international conference on health education, on what it was they were trying to do. This is an easy trap to fall into when terms such as 'health' and 'prevention' can mean such different things to different people. Accordingly, a precise definition of terms was given at the start of this book, not to imply that other views of health and prevention are less valid, but to avoid any ambiguity about what is being discussed (or what is trying to be achieved) and to ensure that terms are used consistently. This final chapter summarizes the observations which have been made so far on each of the seven areas.

11.2. Is an ounce of prevention worth a pound of cure?

On the basis of the analysis in this book the answer appears to be no. The claim that prevention should be vigorously pursued because it will save resources was shown to be true in only isolated cases, and overall to be patently false. What is more important though, and what the preceding analysis has clearly shown, is that such a question is irrelevant. Whether or not prevention saves more than it costs simply does not matter.

It is puzzling that the saving of resources should even be postulated as an objective of prevention since treatment programmes do not have this peculiar expectation attached to them. Rather, it is normally expected that the benefits of treatment will be in terms of healthier people and this will be achieved at some positive net cost. Whether or not this cost is justified (i.e. the programme can be shown to be efficient) will depend on the value attached to these health improvements *vis-à-vis* the value of the opportunity cost. There is no reason why prevention should be viewed in a different way.

A second and related peculiarity concerns the way that the implications of prevention programmes are so often viewed in terms of a lifetime profile of costs and benefits which follow any prevention initiative. There is, of course, nothing wrong with looking at lifetime profiles. What is puzzling is why they are often treated differently in the case of prevention, but not in the case of treatment. With smoking, for example, it is often claimed that economists ought to view smoking as a *good* thing since it kills people and thus reduces the number of elderly in the future who will consume vast amounts of health care resources. The same 'logic' however, rarely seems to be applied to treatment, where success also means more elderly people who consume vast amounts of health care resources. If both prevention and cure produce longer life and/or higher quality of life, then both must be judged by the same criteria.

Throughout this book prevention has been viewed in the same way that treatment programmes or any other economic activities should be viewed. As with these other activities, prevention involves using scarce public or private resources. Consequently, there are always opportunity costs involved. At the same time prevention generates benefits that will almost certainly involve increases in health that are valued for their own sake. The benefits may also include resource savings or productivity gains. Prevention should be judged according to whether the value of all these generated benefits exceeds the opportunity costs.

In only a few cases was it possible, unequivocally, to label any prevention initiative as efficient or inefficient. Among the primary prevention studies, rubella vaccination, fluoridation of water supplies, compulsory use of motorcycle helmets, and banning the sale of non-pasteurized milk were shown to be clearly efficient. Yet all of these involve some form of compulsion. It will be remembered that economic appraisal is never a substitute for decision making, only an aid to it, and the demonstrated efficiency of these compulsory measures provides those who defend freedom of choice with explicit evidence of the price their freedom of choice imposes. Those with the responsibility for deciding whether or not these policies should be pursued must judge whether the value of freedom of choice exceeds this price. The few unequivocally efficient secondary prevention initiatives of Chapter 6 do not involve this degree of compulsion.

For the majority of the studies reviewed here no firm conclusions were possible. The question of efficiency depended either on the values placed on particular intangibles or on some expected improvements in epidemiological or aetiological evidence. It would be unrealistic to expect economic appraisal to provide firmer conclusions when causal relationships are disputed among health professionals. It would be equally unreasonable for economic appraisal to put unequivocal values on intangible costs and benefits when there is little evidence, such as court awards or previous decisions, to indicate what value society places on them. Yet even these inconclusive studies showed the value of the economic approach. In each case provision of the relevant information reduced the valuation problem dramatically and highlighted the values that would be implied whatever decision was taken.

When alternative means of achieving given ends were compared the results provided much valuable cost-effectiveness information. In the case of screening for cancer of the breast, cervix, and colon, for example, it was shown that wider coverage would be more cost-effective than repeated screening of a smaller population. Among different methods of birth control, vasectomy was shown to be most cost-effective. There were also messages for cost-effectiveness even when alternatives were not explicitly compared. The study by Stilwell (1976), for example, suggested that there would almost certainly be more cost-effective ways of preventing tuberculosis than mass BCG vaccination, while Cohen (1982) showed that there were certain to be more cost-effective ways of reducing laboratory acquired infections than the existing Code of Practice.

11.3. Making better use of the cost–benefit approach

The studies which were discussed in Chapters 5 and 6 were selected because by-and-large they applied the principles of economic appraisal appropriately. A favourite teaching technique among health economists in the not too distant past was to select examples of bad economic appraisals (or studies that claimed to be economic appraisals) and ask students to 'spot the errors'. There was no shortage of sample studies to choose from. It is important to note that the quality of most appraisals has improved markedly in recent years and it is becoming increasingly difficult to find the 'howlers' which provided so much amusement to the newly aware students.

The empirical chapters of this book showed that a good application of the cost–benefit approach involves the following:

    1. The study should be broad ranging. The beauty of the principle of

opportunity cost is that nothing can be seen in isolation since everything involves a sacrifice somewhere else. Costing a disease may appear a worthwhile objective, but the cost–benefit approach shows it to be of no value. What matters is what can be done about the disease, what that will cost, and what the sacrifice involved in so doing will be.

2. The study should adopt a societal perspective. In reality, those who make decisions are often concerned only with their own budgets or client populations, and do not care about costs falling on, or benefits accruing to, others. It is not being suggested that such a view is wrong, but by adopting a society-wide approach, those who take the decisions will do so in full awareness of the implications of their chosen action.

3. The study should focus on margins. Decisions to expand or contract a prevention programme are much more common than decisions of the 'do it or don't' variety. Such marginal questions require marginal information. Even questions that are of the 'do or don't' type should not lose sight of margins. In the study by Cohen *et al.* (1983), for example, the marginal cost to the Milk Marketing Board of pasteurizing the additional milk resulting from the ban on the sale of non-pasteurized milk was near zero. Use of the average cost per gallon pasteurized would have been inappropriate and would have overstated the true costs of the ban.

4. The study should include intangibles. As argued above, prevention programmes are unlikely to save resources. The relevance of an analysis limited to a comparison of tangible costs and benefits is dubious. Society does not save resources when it cares for the mentally handicapped, and no cost–benefit appraisal of care for this client group could sensibly be limited to tangible consequences. There is essentially no difference in the case of programmes for prevention. Indeed, the studies reviewed showed that in most cases judgement of efficiency is wholly dependent on the treatment of intangibles.

5. The study should discount future costs and benefits. It is often argued that the process of discounting prejudices all prevention programmes as compared with treatment programmes since the benefits of prevention do not normally arise until long after the costs are incurred. It is certainly true that the greater the delay between the incurring of costs and the realization of benefits the less attractive will the benefit–cost ratio be after discounting, but this owes to the fact that society has a positive rate of time preference. Those who argue that society ought to have a different set of preferences may have a point, but economic appraisal eschews such normative judgements. Failure to discount the future means failure to take account of time preference, and this is simply wrong.

6. The study should assess the importance of assumptions and uncertainties. The only thing that is known about the future is that it is uncertain and no appraisal can be sure that its assumptions will be proved right. What it ought to show, however, is whether or not it matters if any turn out to be wrong. Failure to use sensitivity analysis means failure to demonstrate the robustness of the conclusions. There is a world of difference between something that passes the cost–benefit test regardless of the assumptions and something that passes the test only when certain questionable assumptions hold.

7. Finally, the study should assess equity. This is something rarely seen in the studies reviewed. Economic appraisal is based mainly on efficiency, where a programme passes the test if total benefits exceed total costs. Efficient programmes, however, can have important distributional effects that ought to be considered as well. Those who bear the costs may not be those who gain the benefits and this may be considered unjust. Again, two programmes may be equal in terms of efficiency, but one may benefit the rich while the other benefits the poor, and distributional issues may override efficiency arguments.

11.4. The role of government

Government can play both a direct and an indirect role in the pursuit of prevention. The direct role concerns government expenditures on prevention such as on road safety or on improving the environment. The indirect role concerns all of the ways that governments intervene in the operations of free markets by taxing, subsidizing, and legislating aimed at increasing the demand for and supply of prevention. Economic analysis can be of greatest use in the debate about the nature and extent of the latter role.

By focusing on the maximization of social welfare, subject to other considerations such as equity, economic analysis helps to identify when market imperfections lead to sub-optimal choices being taken. This provides justification for government intervention and helps those who support greater prevention efforts to move away from platitudes and calls from the heart rather than the head.

11.5. The provision of information

When government intervention can be shown to be justified, economic appraisal can also help to identify what forms of intervention can be most cost-effective in achieving the desired objective. The demand studies reviewed here, for example, show that as a means of reducing smoking, tax is a relatively weak policy tool—although it is a good source of government revenue. Studies such as Townsend's (1987) can further identify how taxing cigarettes affects the consumption decisions of different socio-economic groups thus providing useful information to those who choose the 'appropriate' levels of tax. Studies on the demand for alcohol show that beer is less price elastic than wine or spirits thus showing that taxing beer is a less efficient means of reducing consumption than is taxing wine or spirits. The low advertising elasticities of demand for both tobacco and alcohol also provide useful information for policy.

Evidence on the demand for preventive services supplied by health professionals suggests that the scope for increasing consumption by reducing costs to consumers is significant. The evidence on the potential for health education in increasing uptake of preventive services is less conclusive (Fisher 1980), suggesting that subsidizing such services may be the more efficient policy tool.

The supply and demand analyses in this book lend support to the belief that incentives work. An example of how incentives can be used is found in the recently introduced changes in primary care in the UK, where general practitioners are now paid for meeting targets in providing certain preventive services. It is interesting to note that, while incentives to general practitioners are expected to alter supplier behaviour, the UK Government has also claimed that charges to patients for dental check-ups and eye examinations do not have any significant effect on the demand for these services.

The use of incentives need not mean that governments must be seen to be taking on an increased paternalistic role. Rather, it is merely a way of ensuring that consumer and producer decisions are influenced so that they take more account of the consequences of their decisions for health and the health services.

11.6. Understanding preventive behaviour

Economics is a behavioural science and provides an alternative to the socio-psychological approaches to explaining preventive behaviour. Chapter 9 has shown that goods that alter the risk of future illness or injury are different from goods that do not. The demand for prevention is thus different from the demand for other goods in that it is largely derived from the demand for the commodity health, and health is demanded for different reasons than are shoes or haircuts.

11.7. The effect of prevention on the economy

Chapter 2 showed that whereas a hundred years or so ago prevention meant a reduction in infant and child mortality, today it means mainly reducing morbidity and mortality among adults and, especially, increasing the life expectancy of those past retirement age. This has very different implications for the macro-economy. For one thing it means increasing the supply of labour at a time when there is a growing belief that new technology has made full employment in the economy a thing of the past. For another it means that the number of elderly in the population will grow. In addition to increasing the burden of transfer payments in the form of pensions, the elderly consume a larger than proportionate amount of health care. According to the estimate by Gori and Richter (1978) a sudden drop in US mortality rates to those of the second lowest in the industrialized world (a rather unrealistic assumption as the authors admit) would cause US Gross National Product to fall by \$106 billion (1972 prices) and unemployment to rise by 7 million in 20 years. Less dramatic successes for prevention would be far less, if at all, harmful.

Even if prevention were proven to harm the macro-economy, (and evidence to support this is still very contentious), this alone would not provide an argument that prevention was a bad thing. A large and expanding economy is not the only thing of value and it is probable that society would willingly forgo some economic growth potential for these non-financial benefits. Nonetheless, it is better to engage in vigorous pursuit of prevention with full knowledge of all the implications of those policies than to pursue them blindly. There is still a long way to go, but economics is beginning to tease out some of those implications.

11.8. The role of economic policy

Prevention is normally thought of in terms of efforts which are explicitly directed at reducing morbidity and mortality by reducing risk of illness and injury. This book has shown that the possibility of achieving this end by entirely different means may also exist.

The evidence is patchy, but it appears to support the contention that unemployment causes increased morbidity and mortality. If so, then macro-economic policies aimed at reducing unemployment will have the additional benefit of being preventive. The efforts made so far in trying to establish the nature and extent of any causality are laudable. The implications for policy of further efforts in this area are obvious.

11.9. A policy for prevention

The UK National Health Service is often sarcastically called the National Illness Service by those who believe that the prevention potential of the Service has long been ignored in favour of treating the more immediately demanding existing health needs. (The proportion of total NHS expenditure on prevention in 1981 was roughly 5 per cent—Cohen and Henderson 1983.) In many other countries the preventive roles of health services are even more under-used. The message from such critics is that a switch of emphasis (which of course means a switch in resource use) away from treatment and cure and toward prevention is called for.

One interesting feature of the studies in primary prevention reviewed in Chapter 5 was that so few concerned activities carried out within the formal health sector. The identified prevention expenditures for the UK and the US shown in Chapter 10 also showed how the formal health sector plays a limited role in prevention. The Black Report (1982) on inequality in health in the UK did not include measures that involved the NHS among its recommendations on how to reduce the identified inequalities. An efficient prevention strategy may not wish to concentrate too much on initiatives within formal health care sectors, but may want to look much farther afield.

The problem is that going farther afield means involving a host of agencies and organizations whose activities may have an effect on future health, but who may also see themselves as having other, often conflicting, objectives. Even within the public sector such conflicts are evident: the Ministry of Health wants people to eat less saturated fat while the Ministry of Agriculture wants people to eat more butter; the Ministry of Health wants people to smoke less while the Treasury wants the revenue from tobacco duties. Studies may show that increased spending on road safety by local councils will save resources, but because any savings will not accrue to the local councils there may be little incentive for them to do so.

Chapter 10 has shown that as long as responsibility for prevention is badly fragmented and there are few mechanisms to take advantage of the messages emerging from empirical investigations, then an efficient overall prevention policy is unlikely to come about. The efficiency criterion shows where society can potentially benefit because when overall benefits outweigh overall costs the gainers can, in theory, compensate the losers leaving everyone better off, or at least no worse off. If there is no mechanism for seeing that such compensation takes place, and if power currently rests in the hands of the losers, then the programme will not be undertaken.

Chapter 10 also argued for the appointment of a Minister for Prevention, or someone with similar authority. Such a formal position is not strictly necessary, but without some moves to make the national policy for prevention more coherent, such policy will be largely a paper exercise.

Perhaps more important than the above, this book has shown that economics can provide a *framework* within which the efficiency of prevention policy can be considered. The idea behind programme budgeting is that all preventive efforts should be regarded as being part of a single resource management policy since, whatever particular risk factor each initiative addresses, all share the same ultimate goal—more health. Viewing prevention this way means concentrating on the broad objectives of prevention and seeking out information that matches the nature of the objectives and priorities.

11.10. Conclusion

This book suggests that economics has not only contributed quite a lot to prevention and its planning, but that still more can be done. It is perhaps puzzling that economics has not been exploited to a greater degree than it has been. Mooney and Ludbrook (1984) have summarized the main reasons why economic appraisal is not more widely used in health care decision making. They include a lack of awareness of the existence of economic appraisal, a perceived threat to clinical freedom, the nature of the political framework, the current process of decision making, a perceived threat to the professions, practical problems in applying appraisal, and problems in communication. These reasons seem equally applicable in the case of prevention.

Perhaps the main conclusions of this book are very simple yet not widely recognized. Prevention comes in all sorts of shapes, sizes, and guises. It is the responsibility overall of all and yet, at the same time, of none. To those who 'believe in prevention' the message is surely to prove that the benefits of prevention justify the costs; to show where this is the case and to what extent. To the disbelievers, the message is to prove that there are better ways of promoting health. Inevitably, in our view as economists, *some* prevention activities are justified on efficiency grounds and some are not. The message is thus not to show that prevention works, but rather to show which forms of prevention are worthwhile and which are not. As in so many fields of endeavour informed choice is an important objective. It is that objective that economics can promote in determining strategies for prevention.

References

Advisory Committee on Novel and Irradiated Foods (1986). *Report on the safety of irradiated foods.* HMSO, London.

Altman, D.G., Flora, J.A., Fortmann, S.P., and Farquhar, J.W. (1987). The cost-effectiveness of three smoking cessation programs. *American Journal of Public Health,* 77, 162–5.

Andreano, R.L. and McCollum, D.W. (1983). A benefit–cost analysis of amniocentesis. *Social Biology,* 30, 347–73.

Arnould, R.J. and Grabowski, H. (1981). Auto safety regulation: an analysis of market failure. *Bell Journal of Economics,* 12, 27–48.

Atkinson, A.B. and Skegg, J.L. (1973). Anti-smoking publicity and the demand for tobacco in the U.K. *Manchester School of Economics and Social Studies,* 41, 265–82.

Barker, D.J.P. and Rose, G.A. (1979). *Epidemiology in medical practice.* (2nd ed.) Churchill Livingstone, Edinburgh.

Becker, G. (1964). *Human capital.* Columbia University Press, New York.

Becker, M.H. and Maiman, L.A. (1975). Sociobehavioural determinants of compliance with health and medical recommendations. *Medical Care,* 13, 10–24.

Berwick, D.M., Cretin, S., and Keeler, E. (1981). Cholesterol, children and heart disease: an analysis of alternatives. *Pediatrics,* 68, 721–30.

Black Report (1982). *Inequalities in health.* P. Townsend, and N. Davidson, (eds.). Penguin, Harmondsworth.

Blaxter, M. and Patterson, E. (1982). *Mothers and daughters. A three-generational study of health attitudes and behaviour.* Heinemann Educational, London.

Booth, M., Hardman, G., and Hartley, K. (1986). Data note 6. The U.K. alcohol and tobacco industries. *British Journal of Addiction,* 81, 825–30.

Bourgeois, J.C. and Barnes, J.G. (1979). Does advertising increase alcohol consumption? *Journal of Advertising Research,* 19, 21–9.

Brenner, M.H. (1967). Economic change and mental hospitalization, New York State, 1910–1960. *Social Psychiatry,* 2, 180–8.

—— (1973). Fetal, infant, and maternal mortality during periods of economic instability. *International Journal of Health Services,* 3, 145–59.

—— (1977). Health Costs and benefits of economic policy. *International Journal of Health Services,* 7, 581–623.

—— (1979). Mortality and the national economy: A review, and the experience of England and Wales, 1936–76. *Lancet,* ii, 568–73.

British Thoracic and Tuberculosis Association (1975). *Tubercle,* 56, 129.

Bush, J.W., Chen, M.M., and Patrick, D.L. (1973). Health status index in cost effectiveness: analysis of PKU program. In R.L. Berg (ed.) *Health status indexes.* Hospital Research and Education Trust, Chicago, 172–94.

Chamberlain, J. *et al.* (1975). Validity of clinical examination and mammography as screening tests for breast cancer. *Lancet,* ii, 1026–30.

Chang, H.S. and Hsing, Y. (1980). Effect of mortality reductions on economic growth in the United States, 1940–75. *Social Science and Medicine*, **14C**, 237–42.

Chen, Y., Li, W., and Yu, S. (1986). Influence of passive smoking on admissions for respiratory illness in early childhood. *British Medical Journal*, **293**, 303–6.

Cohen, D.R. (1981). *Prevention as an economic good*. Health Economics Research Unit, Discussion Paper no. 02/81, University of Aberdeen, Aberdeen.

—— (1982). The Howie Code: is the price of safety too high? *Journal of Clinical Pathology*, **35**, 101–7.

—— (1983). Health education as a demand concept. *International Journal of Social Economics*, **10**, 52–62.

—— (1984a). Utility model of preventive behaviour. *Journal of Epidemiology and Community Health*, **38**, 61–5.

—— (1984b). *Economic consequences of a non-smoking generation*. Health Economics Research Unit, Discussion Paper no. 06/84, University of Aberdeen, Aberdeen.

—— and Moir, A. (1981). *Who does what in prevention?* Health Economics Research Unit, Discussion Paper no. 09/81, University of Aberdeen, Aberdeen.

—— Porter, I.A., Reid, T.M.S., Sharp, J.C.M., Forbes, G.I., and Paterson, G.M. (1983). A cost–benefit study of milk-borne salmonellosis. *Journal of Hygiene*, **19**, 17–23.

—— and Henderson, J.B. (1983). *A Minister for Prevention: an initiative in health policy*. Health Economics Research Unit, Discussion Paper no. 02/83, University of Aberdeen, Aberdeen.

—— and Henderson, J.B. (1984a). Co-ordinating prevention. *Effective Health Care*, **2**, 7–13.

—— and Henderson, J.B. (1984). No strategy for prevention. In A. Harrison and J. Gretton (eds) *Health Care U.K. 1984: an economic, social, and policy audit*. CIPFA, London, pp. 63–8.

—— and Mooney, G.H. (1984). Prevention goods and hazard goods: a taxonomy. *Scottish Journal of Political Economy*, **31**, 92–9.

Comanor, W.S. and Wilson, T.A. (1974). *Advertising and market power*. Harvard University Press, Cambridge, Mass.

Conway, S.P. (1990). BCG vaccination in children. *British Medical Journal*, **301**, 1059–60.

Cretin, S. (1977). Cost/benefit analysis of treatment and prevention of myocardial infarction. *Health Services Research*, **12**, 174.

Cropper, M.L. (1977). Health, investment in health, and occupational choice. *Journal of Political Economy*, **86**, 1273–94.

Cullis, J.G. and West, P.A. (1979). *The economics of health: an introduction*. Martin Robertson, Oxford.

Culyer, A.J. (1976). *Need and the National Health Service*. Martin Robertson, London.

Culyer, A.J. (ed.) (1983). *Health indicators*. Martin Robertson, Oxford.

Cumper, G. (1982). Social and organisational constraints on health development. *Journal of Tropical Medicine and Hygiene*, **58**, 47–55.

Davies, G.N. (1973). Fluoride in the prevention of caries; a tentative cost–benefit analysis. *British Dental Journal*, **135**, 79–82, 173–4, 233–5, 293–7, 333–6.

Day, N.E. (1989). Screening for cancer of the cervix. *Journal of Epidemiology and Community Health*, **43**, 103–6.

Department of Health (1990). *Blood cholesterol testing: report by the Standing Medical Advisory Committee*. Department of Health, London.

Department of Health (1991). *The health of the nation*. Cm1523, HMSO, London.

Department of Health and Social Security (1977). *Prevention and health*. HMSO, London.

—— (1978). *Code of practice for the prevention of infection in clinical laboratories and post-mortem rooms (Howie Code)*. HMSO, London.

—— (1979). *Report of a working group on screening for open neural tube defects*. HMSO, London.

Doessel, D.P. (1980). *Cost-benefit analysis and water fluoridation; An Australian study*. Health Research Project, Research Monograph 1, Australian National University, Canberra.

Doll, R. (1983). Prospects for prevention. *British Medical Journal*, **280**, 445–53.

Eddy, D.M. (1981). Appropriateness of cervical cancer screening. *Gynecologic Oncology*, **12**, S168–87.

—— (1981). Screening for cancer in adults. In *The value of preventive medicine*. Pitman (Ciba Foundation Symposium 110), London, 88–103.

Ermisch, J. (1983). *The political economy of demographic change*. Heinemann Educational Books for the Policy Studies Institute, London.

Feldstein, M.S., Piot, M.A., and Sundaresan, K.J. (1973). Resource allocation model for public health planning: a case study of tuberculosis control. WHO Geneva (Supplement to Vo. 48 of the *Bulletin of the World Health Organisation*).

Fidler, P.E. (1977). A comparison of treatment patterns and cost for a fluoride and non-fluoride community. *Community Health*, **9**, 103–13.

Fine, P.E.M. and Clarkson, J.A. (1986). Individual versus public priorities in the determination of optimal vaccination policies. *American Journal of Epidemiology*, **124**, 1012–20.

Fisher, L.A. (1980). *Effectiveness and efficiency in health education*. Health Economics Research Unit, Discussion Paper no. 09/80, University of Aberdeen, Aberdeen.

Forbes, J.F. and McGregor, A. (1987). Male unemployment and cause-specific mortality in postwar Scotland. *International Journal of Health Services*, **17**, 233–40.

Forester, T.H., McNown, R.F., and Singell, L.D. (1984). A cost–benefit analysis of the 55 m.p.h. speed limit. *Southern Economic Journal*, **50**, 631–41.

Fuchs, V.R. (1972). Health care and the U.S. economic system. *Millbank Memorial Fund Quarterly*, **50**, 211–37.

Fujii, E.T. (1980). The demand for cigarettes: further empirical evidence and its implications for public policy. *Applied Economics*, **12**, 479–89.

Garfinkel, L., Auerbach, O., and Joubert, L. (1985). Involuntary smoking and lung cancer: a case control study. *Journal of the National Cancer Institute*, **75**, 463–9.

Geiser, E.E. and Menz, F.C. (1976). The effectiveness of public dental care programs. *Medical Care*, **14**, 189–98.

Glass, N. (1979). Evaluation of health service developments. In K. Lee (ed.) *Economics and health planning*. Croom Helm, London, pp. 100–17.

Godfrey, C. (1986). *Factors influencing the consumption of alcohol and tobacco—A review of demand models*. Centre for Health Economics, Discussion Paper no. 16, University of York, York.

Gori, G.B. and Richter, B.J. (1978). Macroeconomics of disease prevention in the United States. *Science*, **200**, 1123–30.

Goss, J. (1985). The economics of reducing hypertension through reduction of sodium intake. In J.R.G. Butler and D.P. Doessel (eds) *Economics and health 1985*. Proceedings of the seventh Australian conference of health economists. University of New South Wales, Kensington.

Gravelle, H.S.E. and Simpson, P. (1979). *Economic analysis of breast cancer screening.* Paper presented to the UK Health Economists' Study Group, Aberdeen.

Gravelle, H.S.E., Hutchinson, G., and Stern, J. (1981). Mortality and unemployment: a critique of Brenner's time series analysis. *Lancet,* **ii,** 275–9.

Gravelle, H.S.E., Simpson, P.R., and Chamberlain, J. (1982). Breast cancer screening and health service costs. *Journal of Health Economics,* **1,** 185–207.

Grosse, R.N. (1980). Interrelation between health and population: observations derived from field experience. *Social Science and Medicine,* **14C,** 99–120.

Grossman, M. (1972). On the concept of health capital and the demand for health. *Journal of Political Economy,* **80,** 223–55.

—— (1982). The demand for health after a decade. *Journal of Health Economics,* **1,** 1–3.

Gudex, C. (1986). *QALYs and their use by the health service.* Centre for Health Economics, Discussion Paper no. 20, University of York, York.

Guzick, D.S. (1978). Efficacy of screening for cervical cancer: a review. *American Journal of Public Health,* **68,** 125–34.

Hagard, S. and Carter, F.A. (1976). Preventing the birth of infants with Down's syndrome: a cost–benefit analysis. *British Medical Journal,* **i,** 753–6.

Haiart, D.C., McKenzie, L., and Henderson, J.B. (1990). Mobile breast screening: factors affecting uptake, efforts to increase response and acceptability. *Public Health,* **104,** 239–47.

Hamilton, J.K. (1972). The demand for cigarettes: advertising, the health scare, and the cigarette advertising ban. *Review of Economics and Statistics,* **56,** 401–11.

Hartz, A.J. *et al.* (*1987*). The association of smoking with clinical indicators of altered sex steroids—a study of 50,145 women. *Public Health Reports,* **102,** 254–9.

Henderson, J.B. (1982). An economic appraisal of the benefits of screening for open spina bifida. *Social Science and Medicine,* **16,** 545–60.

—— (1985). Appraising options: a practical guide. *Hospital and Health Services Review,* **81,** 286–91.

—— McKenzie, L., Haiart, D.C.H., and Moffat, W. (1988). *Uptake of breast cancer screening: an economic demand analysis of attendance rates at a mobile mammography service.* Health Economics Research Unit, Discussion Paper no. 03/88, University of Aberdeen, Aberdeen.

HM Treasury (1980). The change in revenue from an indirect tax change. *Economic Trends,* March, 97–107.

—— (1991). *Economic appraisal in central government: a technical guide for government departments.* HMSO, London.

House of Commons (*Hansard*) (1986). **91,** Col. 527.

Ippolito, P.M. (1981). Information and the life cycle consumption of hazardous goods. *Economic Inquiry,* **19,** 529–58.

Ippolito, P.M. and Ippolito, R.A. (1984). Measuring the value of life saving from consumer reactions to new information. *Journal of Public Economics,* **25,** 53–81.

Jackson, D. (1987). Has the decline of dental caries in English children made waterfluoridation both unnecessary and uneconomic? *British Dental Journal,* Mar. 7, 170–3.

Johnson, J. (1980). Advertising and the aggregate demand for cigarettes. A comment. *European Economic Review,* **14,** 117–25.

Jones-Lee, M.W., Hammerton, M., and Philips, P.R. (1985). The value of safety: results of a national sample survey. *Economic Journal,* **95,** 49–72.

Joyce, T.J., Grossman, M., and Goldman, F. (1989). An assessment of the benefits of air pollution control: the case of infant death. *Journal of Urban Economics,* **25,** 32–51.

Kahneman, D. and Tversky, A. (1979). Prospect theory: an analysis of decision under risk. *Econometrica*, **47**, 263–89.

Keeler, E.B., Brook, R.H., Goldberg, G.A., Kamberg, C.J., and Newhouse, J.P. (1985). How free health care reduced hypertension in the health insurance experiment. *Journal of the American Medical Association*, **254**, 1926–31.

Knapp, M. (1984). *The Economics of Social Care*. Macmillan, Basingstoke.

Koopmanschap, M.A., Lubbe, K.T., van Oortmarssen, G.J., van Agt, H.M., van Ballegooijen, M., and Habbema, J.D.F. (1990). Economic aspects of cervical cancer screening. *Social Science and Medicine*, **30** (10), 1081–7.

Kristein, M. M. (1980). The economics of screening for colo-rectal cancer. *Social Science and Medicine*, **14**, 274–84.

Lambin, J.J. (1975). *Advertising, competition and market conduct in oligopoly over time*. Elsevier North Holland, Amsterdam.

Lancaster, K. (1966). A new approach to consumer theory. *Journal of Political Economy*, **74**, 132–57.

Lau, H. (1975). Cost of alcoholic beverages as a determinant of alcohol consumption. In R.J. Gibbins *et al.* (eds) *Research advances in alcohol and drug problems 2*. John Wiley & Sons, New York, pp. 211–45.

Lave, C.A. (1985). Speeding, coordination and the 55 mph limit. *American Economic Review*, **75**, 1159–64.

Law, M.R., Frost, C.D., and Wald, N.J. (1991). By how much does dietary salt reduction lower blood pressure? (iii) Analysis of data from trials of salt reduction. *British Medical Journal*, **302**, 819–24.

Layde, P.M., von Allmen, S.D., and Oakley, G.P. (1979). Material serum alphafetoprotein screening: a cost–benefit analysis. *American Journal of Public Health*, **69**, 566–72.

Leu, R.E. (1984). Anti-smoking publicity, taxation, and the demand for cigarettes in the United States. *Journal of Health Economics*, **3**, 1–14.

Lewitt, E.M., Coate, D., and Grossman, M. (1981). The effects of government regulation on teenage smoking. *Journal of Law and Economics*, **24**, 545–70.

Loehman, E. *et al.* (1979). Distributional analysis of regional benefits and costs of air quality control. *Journal of Environmental Economics and Management*, **6**, 222–43.

Logan, A.G., Milne, B.J., Achber, C., Campbell, W.P., and Haynes, R.B. (1981). Cost-effectiveness of a worksite hypertension treatment program. *Hypertension*, **3**, 211–18.

Luce, B.R. and Schweitzer, S.O. (1978). The economic costs of smoking-induced illness. *National Institute of Drug Abuse Research Monograph Series*, **17**, 221–9.

McAvinchey, I.D. (1982). *Unemployment and mortality: some aspects of the Scottish case, 1950–78*. Health Economics Research Unit, Discussion Paper no. 10/82, University of Aberdeen, Aberdeen.

McGuinness, T. (1980). An econometric analysis of total demand for alcoholic beverages in the U.K., 1956–75. *Journal of Industrial Economics*, Sept., 85–109.

McGuinness, T. and Cowling, K. (1975). Advertising and the aggregate demand for cigarettes. *European Economic Review*, **6**, 311–28.

McKeown, T. (1979). *The role of medicine: dream, mirage or nemesis?* (2nd edn) Basil Blackwell, Oxford.

Medical Research Council (1972). BCG and vole bacillus vaccines in the prevention of tuberculosis in adolescents and in early adult life: Fourth report to the MRC by its tuberculosis vaccines clinical trials committee. *Bulletin of the World Health Organisation*, **46**, 371–85.

Metra Consulting Group Ltd (1979). *The relationship between total cigarette advertising and total cigarette consumption in the U.K.* Metra Consulting Group, London.

Mole, R.H. (1976). Accepting risks for other people. *Proceedings of the Royal Society of Medicine,* **69,** 107–13.

Mooney, G.H. (1977). *The valuation of human life.* Macmillan, London.

—— (1982). Breast cancer screening: a study in cost-effectiveness analysis. *Social Science and Medicine,* **16,** 1277–83.

—— Russell, E.M. and Weir, R.D. (1986). *Choices for health care: a practical introduction to the economics of health provision.* (2nd edn) Macmillan, Basingstoke.

Swerdlow, A.J. (1987). 150 years of Registrar Generals' medical statistics. *Population Trends,* 20–6.

Taylor, P. (1984). *Smoke ring: the politics of tobacco.* The Bodley Head, London.

Thaler, R. and Rosen, S. (1976). The value of saving a life: evidence from the labor market. In N.E. Terleckyj (ed.) *Household production and consumption: studies in wealth and income no. 40.* National Bureau of Economic Research, Columbia University Press, New York.

Tobacco Advisory Council (1981). *Advertising controls and their effects on total cigarette consumption.* TAC, London.

Tobin, M.V. *et al.* (1987). Cigarette smoking and inflammatory bowel disease. *Gastroenterology,* **93,** 316–21.

Townsend, J.L. (1987). Cigarette tax, economic welfare, and social class patterns of smoking. *Applied Economics,* **19,** 355–65.

Trussell, J.T. (1974). Cost *versus* effectiveness of different birth control methods. *Population Studies,* **28,** 85–106.

Tucker, D. (1982). *Tobacco: an international perspective.* Euromonitor Publications, London.

Twaddle, A.C. (1974). The concept of health status. *Social Science and Medicine,* **8,** 29–38.

US Department of Health, Education, and Welfare, Public Health Service (1964). *Smoking and health: report of the Advisory Committee to the Surgeon General,* US Government Printing Office, Washington.

US Department of Health and Human Services (1980). *Promoting health, preventing disease: objectives for the nation.* Public Health Service, Washington.

Wagstaff, A. (1985). Time-series analysis of the relationship between unemployment and mortality: a survey of econometric critiques and replications of Brenner's studies. *Social Science and Medicine,* **21,** 985–96.

Wald, N.J., Nanchahal, K., Thompson, S.G., and Cuckle, H.S. (1986). Does breathing other people's tobacco smoke cause lung cancer? *British Medical Journal,* **293,** 1217–22.

Walsh, B.M. (1982). The demand for alcohol in the U.K., a comment. *Journal of Industrial Economics,* **30,** 439–46.

Warner, K.E. (1977). The effects of the anti-smoking campaign on cigarette consumption. *American Journal of Public Health,* **67,** 645–50.

Waterson, M.J. (1981). *Advertising and alcohol abuse.* The Advertising Association, London.

Weisbrod, B.A. (1964). Collective-consumption services of individual consumption goods. *Quarterly Journal of Economics,* **78,** 471–7.

Williams, A. (1985). Economics of coronary artery bypass grafting. *British Medical Journal,* **291,** 326–9.

Rosenstock, I.M. (1966). Why people use health services. *Millbank Memorial Fund Quarterly*, **78**, 94–124.

Royal College of Physicians (1962). *Smoking and health*. Pitman Medical, London.

—— (1977). *Smoking or health*. Pitman Medical, London.

—— (1983). *Health or smoking*. Pitman, London.

Russell, L.B. (1986). *Is prevention better than cure?* The Brookings Institution, Washington.

Russell, M.A.H. (1973). Changes in cigarette price and consumption by men in Britain, 1946–71: a preliminary analysis. *British Journal of Preventive and Social Medicine*, **27**, 1–7.

—— Wilson, C., Taylor, C., and Baker, C.D. (1979). Effect of general practitioner advice against smoking. *British Medical Journal*, **2**, 234–5.

Sackett, D.L. and Torrance, G.W. (1978). The utility of different health states as perceived by the general public. *Journal of Chronic Diseases*, **31**, 697–704.

Saffer, H. and Grossman, M. (1986a). *Endogenous drinking age laws and highway mortality rates of young drivers*. National Bureau of Economic Research Working Paper No. 1982, Cambridge, Mass.

—— (1986b). *Beer taxes, the legal drinking age, and youth motor vehicle fatalities*, National Bureau of Economic Research Working Paper No. 1914, Cambridge, Mass.

Samuelson, P.A. (1976). *Economics*. McGraw-Hill, Tokyo.

Schelling, T.C. (1968). The life you save may be your own. In S.B. Chase (ed.) *Problems in public expenditure analysis*. Brookings Institution, Washington

Schmalensee, R. (1972). *The economics of advertising*. Elsevier North Holland, Amsterdam.

Schoenbaum, S.C., Hyde, J.N., Bartoshesky, L., and Crampton, K. (1976). Benefit-cost analysis of rubella vaccination policy. *New England Journal of Medicine*, **294**, 306–10.

Schweitzer, S.O. (1974). Cost-effectiveness of early detection of disease. *Health Services Research*, **9**, 22–32.

Shapiro, S., Venet, W., Strax, P., Venet, L. and Roeser, R. (1982). Ten- to fourteen-year effect of screening on breast cancer mortality. *Journal of the National Cancer Institute*, **69**, 349–55.

Smith, R. (1981). Medicine and the media. *British Medical Journal*, **282**, 1147.

Stafford, E.M., Jackson, P.R., and Banks, M.H. (1980). Employment, work involvement and mental health in less qualified young people. *Journal of Occupational Psychology*, **53**, 291–304.

Stason, W.B. and Weinstein, M.C. (1977). Allocation of resources to manage hypertension. *New England Journal of Medicine*, **296**, 732–9.

Stilwell, J.A. (1976). Benefits and costs of the schools' BCG vaccination programme. *British Medical Journal*, **1**, 1002–4.

Stjernfeldt, M., Berglund, K., Lindsten, J., and Ludvigsson, J. (1986). Maternal smoking during pregnancy and risk of childhood cancer. *Lancet*, **1**, 1350–2.

Stone, R. (1945). The analysis of market demand. *Journal of the Royal Statistical Society*, **1208**, 286–382.

Sugden, R. (1980). Altruism, duty and the welfare state. In N. Timms (ed.) *Social welfare: why and how?* Routledge and Kegan Paul, London.

Sugden, R. and Williams, A. (1978). *The principles of practical cost-benefit analysis*. Oxford University Press, Oxford.

Sumner, M.T. (1971). The demand for tobacco in the U.K. *The Manchester School*, **39**, 23–36.

Swerdlow, A.J. (1987). 150 years of Registrar Generals' medical statistics. *Population Trends*, 20–6.

Taylor, P. (1984). *Smoke ring: the politics of tobacco*. The Bodley Head, London.

Thaler, R. and Rosen, S. (1976). The value of saving a life: evidence from the labor market. In N.E. Terleckyj (ed.) *Household production and consumption: studies in wealth and income no. 40*. National Bureau of Economic Research, Columbia University Press, New York.

Tobacco Advisory Council (1981). *Advertising controls and their effects on total cigarette consumption*. TAC, London.

Tobin, M.V. *et al.* (1987). Cigarette smoking and inflammatory bowel disease. *Gastroenterology*, **93**, 316–21.

Townsend, J.L. (1987). Cigarette tax, economic welfare, and social class patterns of smoking. *Applied Economics*, **19**, 355–65.

Trussell, J.T. (1974). Cost *versus* effectiveness of different birth control methods. *Population Studies*, **28**, 85–106.

Tucker, D. (1982). *Tobacco: an international perspective*. Euromonitor Publications, London.

Twaddle, A.C. (1974). The concept of health status. *Social Science and Medicine*, **8**, 29–38.

US Department of Health, Education, and Welfare, Public Health Service. (1964). *Smoking and health: report of the Advisory Committee to the Surgeon General*. US Government Printing Office, Washington.

US Department of Health and Human Services (1980). *Promoting health, preventing disease: objectives for the nation*. Public Health Service, Washington.

Wagstaff, A. (1985). Time-series analysis of the relationship between unemployment and mortality: a survey of econometric critiques and replications of Brenner's studies. *Social Science and Medicine*, **21**, 985–96.

Wald, N.J., Nanchahal, K., Thompson, S.G., and Cuckle, H.S. (1986). Does breathing other people's tobacco smoke cause lung cancer? *British Medical Journal*, **293**, 1217–22.

Walsh, B.M. (1982). The demand for alcohol in the U.K., a comment. *Journal of Industrial Economics*, **30**, 439–46.

Warner, K.E. (1977). The effects of the anti-smoking campaign on cigarette consumption. *American Journal of Public Health*, **67**, 645–50.

Waterson, M.J. (1981). *Advertising and alcohol abuse*. The Advertising Association, London.

Weisbrod, B.A. (1964). Collective-consumption services of individual consumption goods. *Quarterly Journal of Economics*, **78**, 471–7.

Williams, A. (1985). Economics of coronary artery bypass grafting. *British Medical Journal*, **291**, 326–9.

—— (1987). Screening for risk of CHD: is it a wise use of resources? In M. Oliver, M. Ashley-Miller, and D. Wood (eds) *Screening for risk of coronary heart disease*. John Wiley and Sons, Chichester, 97–106.

Witt, S.F. and Pass, C.L. (1981). The effects of health warnings and advertising on the demand for cigarettes. *Scottish Journal of Political Economy*, **28**, 86–91.

World Health Organisation. (1958). Constitution of the World Health Organisation, Annex 1. *The first ten years of the World Health Organisation*. Geneva.

Yule, B.F., Forbes, G.I., MacLeod, A.F., and Sharp, J.C.M. (1986). *The costs and benefits of preventing poultry-borne salmonellosis in Scotland by irradiation*. Health Economics Research Unit, Discussion Paper no. 05/86, Aberdeen.

Author index

169

Subject index